JOHN CLARK

TMPK THE

MEAL

PREP

KING

PREP

YOUR-

SELF

SLIM

100 time-saving recipes
all under 500 calories

MICHAEL **MJ** JOSEPH

MICHAEL JOSEPH

UK | USA | Canada | Ireland | Australia
India | New Zealand | South Africa

Michael Joseph is part of the Penguin Random House group of companies
whose addresses can be found at global.penguinrandomhouse.com

The authorized representative in the EEA is Penguin Random House Ireland,
Morrison Chambers, 32 Nassau Street, Dublin D02 YH68

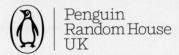

Penguin
Random House
UK

First published 2022
001

Copyright © The Meal Prep King Ltd, 2022
Photography copyright © Jamie Orlando Smith, 2022

The moral right of the author has been asserted

Set in Neutraface
Design and Art Direction by Smith & Gilmour Ltd
Food Stylist: Phil Mundy
Props Stylist: Hannah Wilkinson
Colour reproduction by Altaimage Ltd
Printed and bound by Livonia Print, Latvia

A CIP catalogue record for this book is available from the British Library

ISBN: 978-0-241-55811-9

www.greenpenguin.co.uk

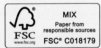

MIX
Paper from
responsible sources
FSC® C018179

Penguin Random House is committed to a
sustainable future for our business, our readers
and our planet. This book is made from Forest
Stewardship Council® certified paper.

CONTENTS

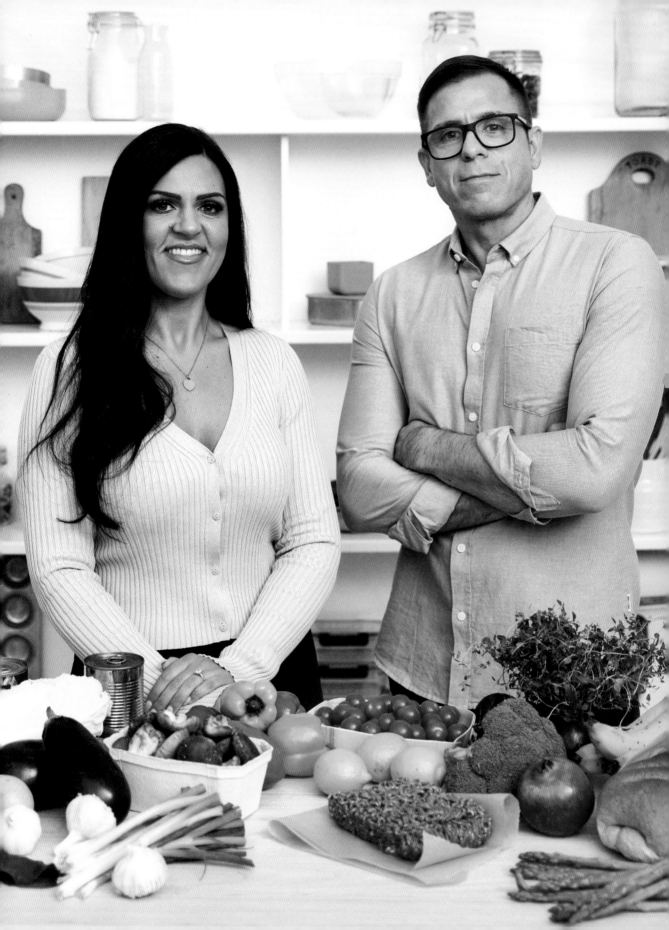

INTRODUCTION

Hello and welcome to the brand-new cookbook.

It's been amazing to see so many of you change your lives with the first book – ditching the fad diets and regaining control. The before and after pictures I get sent on a daily basis showing your results have been nothing short of incredible. You have been asking for more recipes, so we have put together this new cookbook with the most requested recipes from our posts and some new ones – and they are all under 500 calories. We hope you love this cookbook as much as the first one.

When people think about losing weight, they assume they will be restricted to bland, boring foods that they literally dread eating. With this cookbook, we show you this simply isn't true; you can eat what you like, within reason of course. Charlotte and I have lost a combined 15 stone and we eat everything from spinach to salmon, burgers to pizza. Our aim is to help you achieve results that are both practical and sustainable, and we are living proof that what we do works.

You may be starting out on your weight-loss journey for the very first time, or you may be one of those people who have been yo-yo dieting for years, in search of something more long-lasting. When the weight just doesn't seem to stay off, it can leave you desperate and confused about what works and what doesn't – and often leads you ultimately back to the fad diet or plan that failed you the first time round. You are not alone; I have been there and so has Charlotte – we have tried them all.

We hate the word 'diet' as it signals there's an end, when in reality there is no end to needing food! Instead, it's about creating a lifestyle that lasts a lifetime; 'lifestyle' is a term we would much rather emphasize. Weight loss is as much about mindset as it is the foods you eat and we aim to give you top tips to help you achieve long-lasting results.

Let's get started!
John

GETTING STARTED

There's a few 'need to knows' when starting your meal prep journey, especially as understanding why meal prepping works helps to keep you on the right track.

How to lose weight

In basic terms, the way to lose weight is to create a 'calorie deficit' – a reduction of calories consumed relative to the number of calories your body needs to maintain your current body weight. In a deficit, your body is burning off more calories than you are taking in and so has to turn to its energy stores – any fat you might be carrying – to fuel your day-to-day activities. And the more active you are, the more calories your body will burn, increasing the deficit.

For example, to lose 1lb of fat, you need to create a caloric deficit of 3,500 calories over a week. So, let's say you want to lose 1lb a week. You divide the number 3,500 by 7 and that equates to 500. So, your body needs to be consuming 500 calories less per day than it uses. The result is healthy sustainable weight loss.

A deficit can be achieved in a number of ways: firstly, by simply eating less calories with no change in activity levels; secondly, by using exercise alone to create a calorific deficit and keeping your calorie intake at maintenance level; or, my third and favourite way, by combining the two together.

Modestly increasing exercise at the same time as decreasing calories promotes a great routine for both body and mind which is sustainable long term. If you can't get to a gym that's fine – just aim to increase the amount of activity you do. Walking is a great alternative to the gym. Charlotte and I use walking as a way to get quality time together – going out for a stroll gives us time to talk about things and it's quite therapeutic. Those of you who see us on social media will notice we walk quite often. It's also great if you want that extra treat: leave the car at home and walk to the shop instead. If you're walking, you'll feel you've earned it.

How many calories should I be eating to lose weight?

In order to work out roughly how many calories you should be eating each day, you need to work out your total daily energy expenditure (TDEE). While some people may be able to lose weight by restricting their intake to 2,000 calories a day, others will need to reduce their intake a little further. This is where a simple equation will help. Once you have calculated your expenditure, you can go ahead and plan your delicious meals for the week. So let's get started.

Step 1:

To find your TDEE, you need to start by first estimating your basal metabolic rate (BMR). Your BMR is an estimate of how many calories your body burns at rest. The easiest way to work this out is to use an online calculator, or you can punch in the numbers if you wish! This is the most popular equation (Mifflin-St Jeor):

MEN	WOMEN
10 × weight (kg) + 6.25 × height (cm) − 5 × age (years) + 5	10 × weight (kg) + 6.25 × height (cm) − 5 × age (years) − 161

Step 2:

Once you have your BMR, you need to factor in how much activity you do: the more you move, the more calories you expend, and the more food you can plan into your meal prep week. Decide, honestly, which activity level in the chart below best describes you and multiply your BMR by the figure in the multiplier column – now you have your TDEE.

PHYSICAL ACTIVITY LEVEL (PAL)	MULTIPLIER	DESCRIPTION
Mostly inactive	1.2	Mainly sitting
Fairly active	1.3	Sitting, some walking, exercise once or twice per week
Moderately active	1.4	Regular walking, or exercise two to three times per week
Active	1.5	Exercise or sport more than three times per week
Very active	1.7	Physically active job or intense daily exercise or sport

Step 3:

Once you know what your total daily energy expenditure should be, decide how much weight you'd like to lose per week and work out how many calories you need to consume per day to meet that target.

To use myself as an example: when I was 22 stone 6 pounds (142.5kg), I used the formula in Step 1 to calculate that my BMR would be 2470. I was then honest with myself about how much exercise I did (I was fairly active) and so I multiplied my BMR by 1.3.

Based on this, my TDEE would have been around 3211 calories for maintenance of my current body weight. However, I wasn't happy with my current weight, and was actually consuming up to 4,500 calories a day and gaining weight. I set my aim to get to 13 stone by losing a couple of pounds a week.

Using the fact that it takes a deficit of 3,500 calories to lose a pound, I calculated that I would need to reduce my caloric intake by 7,000 calories a week, or 1,000 calories a day. As my TDEE was quite high to begin with, this wasn't as difficult as it may first sound.

I started my journey initially by cutting out alcohol completely as it made up a huge proportion of the calories I was consuming. I left my food pretty much as it was, still enjoying takeaways and junk food most days. I was amazed to see I had dropped a stone just by cutting out alcohol. The next part was to polish up my food, and again, the weight began to come off even faster once I began counting calories.

However, after a period of successful weight loss, I hit a plateau as I got smaller and my TDEE decreased – for a month I didn't lose any weight. I recalculated my TDEE based on my new weight and realised that eating 1,000 calories less per day was going to be very tricky – and not advisable. Instead, I reduced my calorie intake by just 500 a day and started going to the gym. Exercise is a way you can create a higher deficit without decreasing calories as much. It worked for me – and does to this day – but as I always say: you don't need the gym or exercise to lose weight. However, it will speed up the process and be beneficial in the long term for overall physical and mental health.

Mixing and matching calories

How and when you choose to consume your calories is entirely your choice. It doesn't matter what time of day you eat – what does matter is the overall calorie intake over a period of time, such as a day or a week.

I eat the second I wake up in the morning; breakfast is one of my favourite meals of the day. However, unlike me, Charlotte isn't a fan of eating in the morning as she can't face food that early. So, she will often skip breakfast and start eating around lunchtime. If you prefer to have more calories at one meal and less at others, that's completely fine. Split your calories up into four meals over the day, or eat fewer meals of larger portions – it really is up to you.

When mixing and matching calories, having a good intake of nutrients is important to ensure your body is getting exactly what it needs to stay healthy. A balanced diet supplies the nutrients your body needs to work effectively, and without these you are more prone to disease and fatigue. Keep this in mind when making food choices and try and include more fruits, vegetables, lean protein sources and wholegrains. Limit highly processed foods, sugary drinks and things like processed meat. Alcohol also can be a huge source of hidden calories, so be mindful of calories consumed on a night out. Remember everything is okay in moderation, but try and make better choices overall.

How to get motivated to start – and keep going

Motivation comes from taking action. We get asked a lot, 'How do you stay motivated?' or are told, 'I want to lose weight, but I just don't have the motivation'. The truth is that when you take action on your goals, motivation will follow. Motivation comes from friends and family telling you how well you look; from the new clothes that you start to fit into; from that sense of achievement we feel when we follow things through – that's when the real motivation kicks in and keeps you going. A lot of people think motivation comes first when in fact it's the action, then the motivation.

Accept that you're going to have bumps and rocky patches along the way. That's a fact. We are all only human, so don't be too hard on yourself if one day you eat too much, or if you have that birthday meal. Treat these occasions as just that: an occasion. Some people will take a day off from calorie counting or making healthier choices and then feel they have failed on their journey. The problem for people wanting to lose weight is when one day turns into a week, a week turns into a month, and then that month turns into a year. There is nothing wrong with having a day or even a week off. It's what we do consistently that dictates our outcome. And this is just all part of the process, so don't be too hard on yourself.

Losing weight is simple but it isn't easy. Balance really is key. Eating a variety of foods will help you live a happier, healthier life. Use this book to plan and create your own lifestyle that's sustainable and allows you to eat foods that you enjoy. After all, we all have to eat every day so there's no point eating foods you have to force down for the sake of it or don't look forward to. We'll help you form new, healthier habits so you can literally have your cake and eat it.

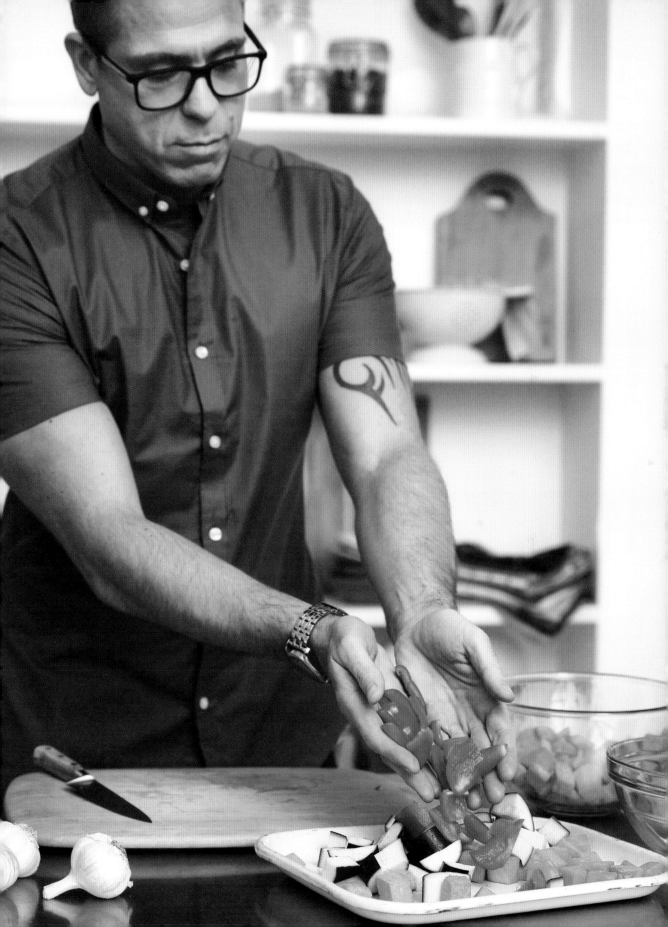

TOP 10 TIPS FOR WEIGHT-LOSS SUCCESS

1 Be honest with yourself

Being honest with yourself about your weight takes a lot of courage. We often lie to ourselves about how much our weight actually bothers us, leading to another year where no progress is made. I was one of those people who always had an excuse – I found every reason I could to procrastinate. But you are different – you have bought this book and are ready to get going. Which is great, as the quicker you are honest with yourself and start your journey the quicker you will see the results. How many times have you said to yourself, 'I'll start my diet on a Monday', 'I'll do it after we have been on holiday', or 'I just have this or that to do first'? Starting now, whatever the day, and breaking the cycle of 'I'll start Monday' really does help.

2 Set yourself realistic goals

Losing ½–2lb per week over a few months is more realistic and achievable for most people than a short burst of crash dieting. But remember, weight will fluctuate in the short term, so take note of the number on the scales over a longer period of time, such as 4–6 weeks. There are going to be some weeks you will lose more than others, so you shouldn't get disheartened if you lose 4lb one week and only ½lb the next. Body measurements are perhaps a better way to gauge progress – I find the best indicator is my clothes: they don't lie.

Ignore what other people are doing and focus on yourself. It's easy to get wrapped up in other people's social media posts, claiming to have lost incredible amounts of weight in a week. Not only is this unrealistic, but it probably isn't true. Remember, you didn't gain weight overnight and you won't lose it overnight either. Be realistic and consistent and you'll reach your goals.

3 Set a date and write it down

Have something to aim for? This could be anything: a wedding, a birthday, a holiday. Set that date in your head, then write down an achievable weight-loss goal. Treat this as your first step to a new you. Setting goals and taking small steps towards that goal really will help you start.

4 Take a selfie

You'll be glad you did. Progress pictures can be extremely helpful over time. I only have two or three images of myself at my biggest. It was a lot easier to avoid photos when I lost my weight back in 2003 as there wasn't a camera phone in everyone's pocket. And I wish I had more images to look back on. So go on . . . take those embarrassing pictures to use as motivation both now and in the future. You won't regret it – trust me.

5 Use the 'power of the coat hanger'

'What does a coat hanger have to do with weight loss?' I hear you ask. One of the many benefits of losing weight is the clothes we fit into when we do. You'll gain confidence and feel a great sense of achievement when you can actually see all your hard work before your eyes.

A very powerful tool I used when I was overweight was to buy an item of clothing a size or two below my current size, which I knew I wouldn't fit into (just yet). I hung it on a door in my bedroom so I'd walk past it every day and be reminded of my goal. Having that mindset every day helps you focus on something achievable. Once I could fit into that item, I'd do the same again, picking an item in a slightly smaller size. I found this trick extremely helpful in losing 9 stone.

6 Never guesstimate your foods

I see so many people guessing calories and then being upset and frustrated when they fail to lose weight, or even gain it. Once people start tracking foods properly, they are amazed at how much they were overeating without even knowing. Weigh almost everything – at least initially until you become familiar with calorie values – and give yourself the confidence that you are eating to the calorie deficit you set yourself.

7 Go to the gym or don't go to the gym

The choice is yours. I am a huge advocate for going to the gym for many reasons, such as mental health, body composition, fitness, routine and just a general sense of wellbeing. However, this isn't essential for weight loss; do the activity you feel comfortable with.

8 Forget the guilt and have that takeaway!

Having a takeaway from time to time is completely fine. I'm partial to getting a pizza or kebab delivered whilst I put my feet up – who isn't? So just have one, and don't try and count the calories. Enjoy it and remember you're only human and losing weight isn't about cutting everything out; it's about balance.

This being said, I also found it extremely beneficial to make my own takeaways from time to time – see my fake-away Friday night pizza (see page 157) or my homemade doner kebab (see page 146). Cooking your own can be fun for the family, can help you stay in control of your calories, and can work out less than a third of the price. The key point here is that you don't have to miss out on anything.

9 Keep a well-stocked fridge

There's something magical about a fridge jam packed with full meal prep containers. When you open the door and all your meals are staring back at you, calorie counted and ready to go, it's extremely motivating.

Knowing you are prepared and in control sets you up to succeed.

You're more likely to eat the foods you've prepared as you've spent the time and effort already – treat that as an investment in yourself to achieve your goals. Food also isn't cheap, but meal prep eliminates the majority of food waste. It's a win–win situation.

10 Remember why you started

This is super important and I'll explain why. When we lose weight, we can quite easily lose focus, which may lead to us put the weight back on. For example, once you have lost a stone, you may revert back to your old lifestyle, gaining it all back plus more, which leads to a vicious cycle of yo-yo dieting. Remembering why you started can be powerful at this point. It may be because you were sick and tired of your clothes not fitting you, you lacked self-confidence, you had health reasons, or it could have been to set a positive example to your children. Whatever it may be, remembering this is a great tool to a long-lasting healthy lifestyle with sustainable results.

It's also worth noting that your reasons for weight loss over time may change. I'm a prime example of this. I set out to lose weight because I was tired of clothes not fitting me, I wanted to attract better-looking girls (I was only 21 at the time), and I was upset with people calling me Fat John. I'd had enough and it was time to change.

Even though I am now at a healthy weight, I've continued meal prepping all these years on because it helps me achieve balance and live a healthier and hopefully longer life. I have learned that you can have everything, just not in excess, and I follow my own advice in this book to this day.

Turn the page for some incredible success stories . . .

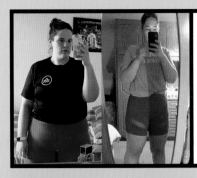

Karen Coffey

The first cookbook helped me so much! Nearly 4 stone lost (and counting) since February 2021! I'm absolutely loving the meals and how simple |everything is. Thank you for helping me and many others on this fitness and weight-loss journey.

I'm absolutely loving the meals and how simple everything is.

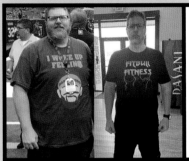

Jimmy Weist

I have battled most of my life – I would lose 20 or so pounds but put it right back on. Following you helped me realize that it is a doable lifestyle while eating what I like. I would get ideas on how to eat what I wanted but smarter portions and healthier options. Your cookbook was so helpful in planning meals and so many tasty recipes. Your real talks and question answering on Instagram are also very inspiring to keep going even if you fall off the wagon. It helped me realize that it's a journey and a lifestyle. Thank you and keep on motivating and creating. I've lost a little over 125lb (9 stone) over the last two years. Slow, smart and steady works and I've been able to keep it off.

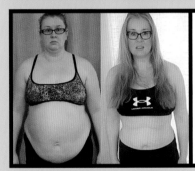

Gemma Bradshaw

The change you see in my before and after pictures is all down to following the ebooks, *The Meal Prep King Plan* book and taking on board all of your advice about calorie counting! I am so excited about the second book, I have no doubt it will be amazing!

The change you see is all down to taking on board all of your advice.

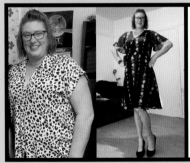

Marissa Chaplin

Buying *The Meal Prep King Plan* book has been an absolute life changer for me. Just before Christmas last year I was at the heaviest I've ever been. I'd tried all the usual ways to lose weight, joining groups, losing a bit, then putting it all back on. Then I came across a post on Instagram about meal prepping and this new book that was coming out. I followed the three week plan in the book and the weight started to disappear week by week. I felt so proud of myself and that gave me the motivation to keep going. Fast forward 10 months and I'm 4 stone lighter and it's the best feeling ever. This journey wouldn't have happened if it wasn't for John and Charlotte and *The Meal Prep King Plan*.

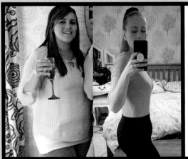

Chantelle Orton

I have lost 6 stone by using your cookbook and it's changed my life and my entire outlook on food. I used to cook convenience foods that were high in fat and calories and quick to prepare. Being a mum to three small children doesn't leave me with much time to cook everyday. Your book has taught me how to calorie count and make small changes that make foods that I love healthier. I'm so ashamed of my before picture but here's my before and after.

Your cookbook has changed my life.

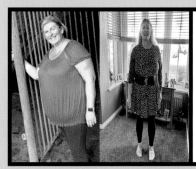

Julie Singleton

Your book has been amazing, with nothing off limits. The recipes are so tasty and healthy. Following your book has stopped me from feeling hungry. I never used to eat a breakfast but now I always do – poppy seed pancakes being my favourite. I make chicken fried rice on a Friday and my husband and son love it. Thanks so much for all your guidance and help in your amazing book. I have followed it for 6 months and have lost 5 stone.

Your book has stopped me from feeling hungry.

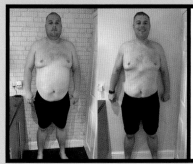

Stephen Orton

A no nonsense way to lose weight, I have lost over 106lb following John's advice, principles and meal ideas. In the past, I have tried endless diets in the attempt to lose weight and was never able to sustain them long enough – I always wanted quick wins. However, John explained that keeping my calories at a decent level didn't leave me feeling hungry or tired, so I stayed consistent and trusted the process and the results are fantastic. I'm now only 42lb away from my target weight!

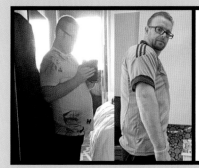

Dave Roberts

It all started when the wife asked me to buy *The Meal Prep King Plan* for Christmas. She followed his Instagram and I became interested when the book arrived and I looked though it. I made BBQ pulled chicken and loved it! We haven't got a big fridge, so we prep three days' worth of meals a week. The book and the Instagram page have helped so much and inspired me to lose weight and exercise more to burn those calories. I look better now in my forties than I did 20 years ago.

I look better now in my 40s than I did 20 years ago.

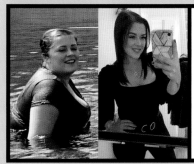

Katie Davies

This book is life changing. Being a shift worker and sometimes finishing late, meal prep has been a life saver. I've lost 4 stone and gone from a size 18 to a size 12. Every recipe I've made from the book has been amazing and I genuinely look forward to trying the next recipes when I batch cook again on Friday.

Being a shift worker and sometimes finishing late, meal prep has been a life saver.

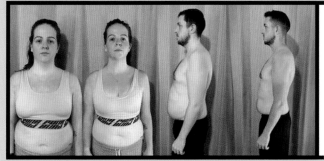

Kate Louise Ellison

Me and my husband Anthony have been following your book since January this year. So far, I have lost 2 stone and my husband 2.5 stone. It's the best thing we have ever done. You made us realize it's not a diet – it's a lifestyle change.

It's not a diet – it's a lifestyle change.

MEAL PREP MADE SIMPLE

Meal prepping is essentially batch cooking. You will save lots of time during the week if you meal prep at a weekend. It will free up those precious hours when you finish work to do the things you enjoy most. But if this doesn't fit your lifestyle, you can choose a day and time that's convenient for you and your family. The beauty is you never have to deliberate over what to eat – no more opening your fridge, seeing it empty and resorting to quick and often unhealthy choices. You will save time, save money and be prepared.

Scaling recipes up

You can scale recipes in this book up. If you really like something, there's nothing to stop you making more of it and freezing extras. If a recipe serves four, feel free to double the ingredients to serve eight, and so on. If you live alone, my advice is to do the recipe as is and freeze the leftover meals for another day, rather than scaling down. Make the fridge and freezer work for you. We have marked with a freezer symbol the meals that will freeze particularly well.

Storing your meal preps

Your meals will last in the fridge for up to three days, with some lasting a little longer, such as the fruit jars. When you have finished cooking, portion out the food into your containers as it will cool down much quicker than if left sitting in the hot pan. Running cold water over pasta and rice will help them cool faster, as will stirring things like soups and stews occasionally as they cool. Try and get your food stored away in the fridge or freezer within 60–90 minutes of cooking, as this will keep nasty bacteria from developing. Make sure you don't leave food sat out for hours.

Saying this, don't be too hasty and put boxes of warm food in your fridge or freezer, as this can raise the temperature inside and mean it isn't as cold as it should be to keep everything chilled or frozen. Your fridge should remain below 5°C and your freezer below -18°C to keep food at its optimum.

It's often better to store accompanying sauces and salad dressings in a separate small container to prevent everything going soggy. It keeps the food fresher, and also means that any sauces that are intended to be served cold can be removed easily before reheating the meal.

Freezing

Freezing is a huge part of the meal prep plan as it means meals can be stored safely and enjoyed weeks later, helping to mix up your diet and decrease food waste. Some foods fare better than others in the freezer, so look out for the freezer symbol for those that freeze well. Just make sure you keep meals that don't freeze well, such as salads, in the fridge and enjoy within three days of preparing. I always have a staple bag of salad in the fridge, so if a freezeable dish is served with salad leaves, I can add those from my fridge stash.

Freeze your food the day it is made in the appropriate portion, so you can just pull a single meal out when you need it. Glass and plastic meal prep containers are freezeable, or you could just use freezer bags if you wish as they can be more space efficient than boxes. Some types can also be washed out and reused.

And one final tip – always label and date the meals you are freezing. However much you think you will remember what a meal is, things can look different when they are frozen and it is easy to be surprised by that curry that turns out to be a pasta sauce! Dating containers also means that meals aren't left in the freezer for years.

Reheating

As with storing food, there are a few food safety tips when it comes to reheating your meals. If a meal is frozen, take it out of the freezer the day before and let it defrost fully in the fridge overnight. Whether you are reheating in the microwave, in the oven or on the hob, always make sure your food is piping hot throughout before eating.

One final, important, thing: never reheat your meal preps more than once. Equally, don't refreeze them either, as the more times you cool and heat food, the higher the risk of food poisoning.

Meal prep kitchen must-haves

There are certain bits of equipment that will help you a lot on your meal prep journey, making the task of prepping feel much easier. Here are my must-haves to help speed up the process:

Non-stick pans Although a certain amount of fat is necessary in cooking, having a set of good-quality non-stick pans helps to reduce the amount of oil or butter needed, reducing calories.

Spray bottle Some low-calorie cooking sprays are known for damaging pans. I like to use a small spray bottle and fill it with oil, creating my own cooking spray that helps oil to go that little bit further. Simply add the spray bottle to a set of kitchen scales and zero before using. Spray your pan, return the bottle to the scales to see the amount used, and calculate the calories.

Glass jars I found out by pure chance that glass preserving jars help fruit stay fresh for longer – we store chopped fruit in them for five days without a problem. Jars are also great for shaking up salad dressings in, and the tiny hotel-buffet-sized jars are useful for storing dressings in, to be added at the last minute, as they will often fit inside your larger meal prep container.

Kitchen scales No meal prep kitchen is complete without a set of kitchen scales. I like digital as these are far more accurate. But remember to have a spare battery on hand – there's nothing worse than when your scales stop working halfway through a meal prep day.

Meal prep storage containers You will need somewhere to store all your meal prep portions. I like to have both glass and plastic meal prep containers. They both have their pros and cons:
Glass meal prep containers are long lasting, easy to clean and they don't stain. They can be used in the oven, microwave and the freezer, making them really versatile. The downside is they can break (but not easily), they are quite heavy if you're taking your meal with you on the go, they don't stack as well as plastic containers, and they can also be more expensive than plastic. This being said, I couldn't live without my glass meal prep containers.
Plastic meal prep containers are cheaper than glass, they are lightweight, and they stack very well. The downside is that you can't put these in the oven and they eventually do wear out.

I would personally recommend having both types of meal prep containers. The amount you will need depends on the amount of food you meal prep and for how many people. Charlotte and I have 20 glass containers and 20 plastic for the week. You also need to consider how many containers you might have stored away in the freezer at any time. It's also worth investing in a few tiny tubs that will fit inside your main container to store any dressings separately.

Space in the freezer A lot of the recipes in this book freeze really well and that's no accident. By storing meals in the freezer you can add more variety to your meal prep plans for the week, and also have plenty ready for the weeks when you might not be able to fit a meal prep day in.

OUR ONE-WEEK MEAL PLAN EXAMPLE

The picture opposite is a typical meal prep week for me and Charlotte – it will keep us going through the working week, and then we cook fresh over the weekend. This isn't all we eat either; depending on daily activities, and any exercise we do, we will add things, such as bread, chocolate, protein bars or shakes etc, to our prepped food. But these meals shown are the bulk of our meals, taking away most of the washing up for the week,

most of the cooking, saving us money and giving us time to do other things.

This is an example that fits our current lifestyle and circumstances; you can try out what we do or create your own plan around your lifestyle, work and family commitments. Meal prep is so adaptable for everyone. It may be that you have a large family so you want to prepare more of the meal preps that will freeze well and take advantage of

BREAKFAST	LUNCH	DINNER	SNACK
Monday			
Breakfast Fruit Jars (page 26)	Thai Turkey Lettuce Wraps (page 87)	TMPK Burger (page 136)	Peanut Butter Cups (page 194)
Tuesday			
Breakfast Fruit Jars (page 26)	Thai Turkey Lettuce Wraps (page 87) OR Spinach, Feta and Pine Nut Pies (page 62)	TMPK Burger (page 136) OR Lamb Kebabs with Root Mash (page 143)	Peanut Butter Cups (page 194)
Wednesday			
Breakfast Fruit Jars (page 26)	Spinach, Feta and Pine Nut Pies (page 62)	Lamb Kebabs with Root Mash (page 143)	Peanut Butter Cups (page 194)
Thursday			
Breakfast Fruit Jars (page 26)	Plum Tomato, Basil and Red Lentil Soup (page 52)	Honey Soy Garlic Chicken with Rice (page 124)	Peanut Butter Cups (page 194)
Friday			
Breakfast Fruit Jars (page 26)	Plum Tomato, Basil and Red Lentil Soup (page 52)	Honey Soy Garlic Chicken with Rice (page 124)	Peanut Butter Cups (page 194)

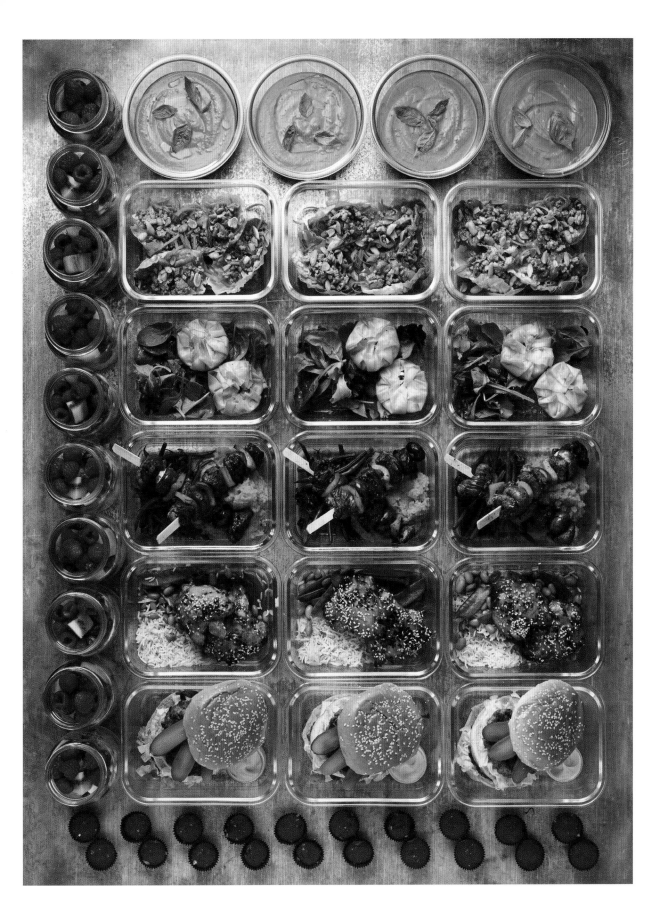

freezer space. You may want to meal prep just lunches or dinners. Or you might find that meal prepping sweet treats and freezing them can be a great way to keep you from overeating. Experiment with the recipes and use our tips to help you build habits that work for your situation.

Why do you meal prep in threes?
I'm glad you've asked.

It's worth explaining how and why we meal prep on a Sunday and for the days that we do. Our meal prep is very specific to us and our lifestyle and here's why.

When I first met Charlotte, she wasn't eating and she was literally starving herself in a last-ditch attempt to lose weight. Charlotte and I don't live together (yet!) so when she went home, I wanted to ensure she was eating as I was genuinely worried about her.

Charlotte would arrive at my house on a Friday evening after work and she would leave first thing in the morning on a Monday after spending the weekend. So, I would make the meals she needed for the week on a Sunday for her to take home. I needed nine main meals, five breakfasts, and five mid-afternoon snacks for Charlotte for the week she wasn't with me – this would provide one breakfast Monday to Friday, one lunch Monday to Friday, one snack Monday to Friday and a dinner Monday to Thursday. Charlotte would then come to my house Friday night and we would cook fresh all weekend.

I worked out Charlotte's TDEE (see pages 6–7) and how many calories she would need roughly over the week given her activity levels, age, sex and goals, and I set to work each and every Sunday prepping meals for us both. I knew this would work for Charlotte as I'd been doing this for years effectively. And I knew she would succeed and trust me if I did it alongside her every week. Charlotte lost 6 stone in 10 months eating this way and I've never seen her as happy.

As I started to post the meal preps on social media, people were so inspired by our story they wanted to see more. My kitchen work top, frustratingly, will only fit meals in sets of three neatly, not four, so meal prep in threes was born. I didn't realize at the time that 'Why do you meal prep in threes?' was to become the most asked question across my social media of nearly two million followers. But this is the honest reason.

However, it came with a very unique benefit we hadn't thought about when we set out. We split the meal prep containers between us, so if one of us likes a meal more than another, that person will have two of those. Let's say we made three portions of meatballs: they are my favourite so I'd have two of those that week and Charlotte would have one portion of those and take two of something else she preferred.

It's a little irregular, but it works out great for us. However, I recognize that many couples might prefer to cook together, so for ease we have kept all the recipes in this book as multiples of two. As most of the meals keep for several days in the fridge or freeze well, you can be as flexible as you like and mix things up. That's the joy of meal prepping – it's easy to make it work for you. Now, on to the recipes!

Shopping List

FRUIT, VEGETABLES AND FRESH HERBS

- [ ] 750g blueberries
- [ ] 10 tangerines
- [ ] 10 kiwis
- [ ] 500g raspberries
- [ ] 1 lime
- [ ] 3 onions
- [ ] 2 red onions
- [ ] 650g carrots
- [ ] 500g swede
- [ ] 400g spinach leaves
- [ ] 1 yellow pepper
- [ ] 16 smallish mushrooms
- [ ] 1 large romaine lettuce or 2 little gem lettuces
- [ ] 2 leaves iceberg lettuce
- [ ] 2 red chillies
- [ ] fresh ginger
- [ ] 2 garlic bulbs
- [ ] 3 spring onions
- [ ] 25g fresh basil
- [ ] 10g fresh rosemary
- [ ] 10g fresh dill
- [ ] 10g fresh chives or parsley

MEAT AND FISH

- [ ] 500g turkey breast mince
- [ ] 8 skinless, bone-in chicken thighs
- [ ] 600g lean beef mince
- [ ] 350g lean lamb

DAIRY AND EGGS

- [ ] butter
- [ ] low-fat margarine
- [ ] low-fat crème fraîche
- [ ] 1 packet feta cheese
- [ ] 1 packet low-fat processed cheese slices

GENERAL

- [ ] 190g smooth peanut butter
- [ ] sesame seeds
- [ ] 50g pine nuts
- [ ] peanuts
- [ ] 120g red lentils
- [ ] 160g rice
- [ ] 1 pouch cooked rice
- [ ] gherkins
- [ ] 1 mini bottle of red wine (187ml)
- [ ] 6 large rectangular sheets filo pastry
- [ ] 6 seeded brioche burger buns
- [ ] bread (to go with your soup)
- [ ] 260g milk or dark chocolate
- [ ] 2 x 400g tins plum tomatoes in juice

STORECUPBOARD

- [ ] American-style yellow mustard
- [ ] ancho chilli flakes
- [ ] coconut oil
- [ ] dark soy sauce
- [ ] ground allspice
- [ ] honey
- [ ] lighter than light mayo
- [ ] low-calorie cooking oil spray
- [ ] olive oil
- [ ] rice vinegar
- [ ] sesame oil
- [ ] sugar
- [ ] Thai red curry paste
- [ ] vegetable stock pots
- [ ] white vinegar
- [ ] salt and pepper

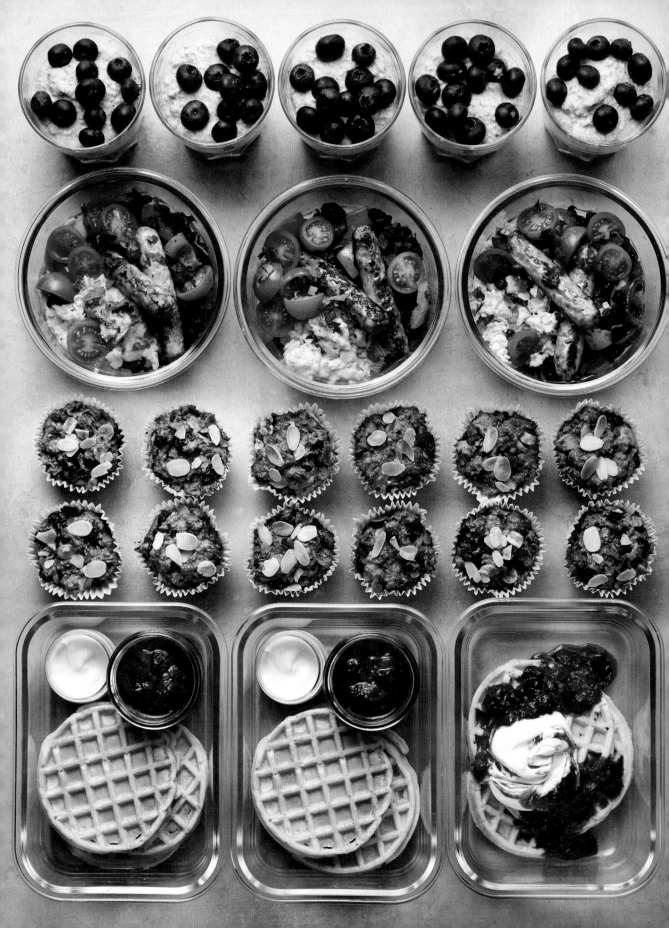

BREAKFAST

410
CALS

TOASTED SEED AND BUCKWHEAT PORRIDGE

PER SERVING | **410** CALS | **15G** PROTEIN | **14G** FAT | **55G** CARBS

prep *cook*
5 MINS 15 MINS

SERVES 4

For the mix:
80g buckwheat groats
    (kasha)
60g mixed seeds
    (buy a bag of mixed
    seeds, or make it up
    from pumpkin seeds,
    sunflower seeds, sesame
    seeds, linseed, etc)
160g whole rolled oats
a pinch of salt

*For one bowl of porridge
(scale up as necessary):*
70g porridge mix
    (see above)
150ml semi-skimmed milk
    or unsweetened almond
    milk (roasted, if wished)
1 tsp honey

tip

*The dry mix for this
porridge keeps well in an
airtight container, so you
could double the recipe
and have a few batches
ready to go when you
need porridge in a hurry.*

*A creamy, comforting porridge, with toasty flavours from
the seeds and buckwheat. You can buy buckwheat groats
from your local Polish shop, or you will find them in the
international aisle of many supermarkets.*

1 To make the porridge mix, preheat the oven to 180°C fan.
Tip the buckwheat groats and mixed seeds onto a large, lipped
baking tray and bake for 5 minutes. Mix them around, add the
oats and bake for another 3 minutes, then leave everything
to cool. Stir in a good pinch of salt. You can store this mixture
in an airtight container until ready to make your porridge.

2 To make the porridge, put 70g of the mix per person into
a small saucepan and add 150ml milk per person. Heat very
gently over a low heat, stirring, until the oats are cooked and
tender. This should take about 5 minutes. If the porridge is
becoming too thick before the oats are cooked, add a splash
of water – 50ml or thereabouts, depending on how runny
you want it.

3 Tip the porridge into a bowl and drizzle the honey over
to serve.

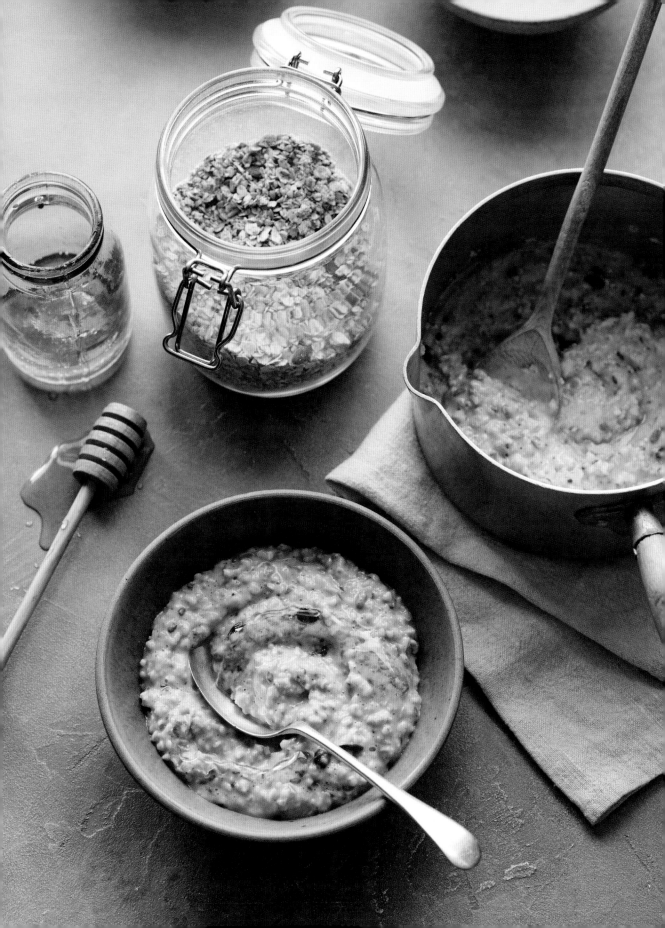

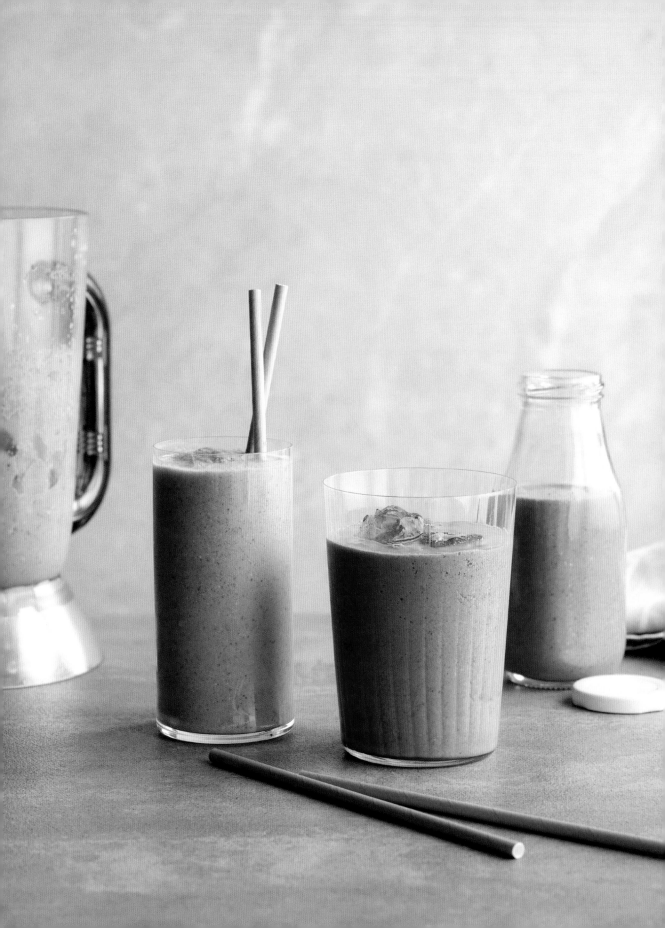

ALMOND AND PRUNE BREAKFAST SHAKE

PER SERVING | **15G** PROTEIN | **16G** FAT | **32G** CARBS

 342 CALS prep 5 MINS

Prunes are a brilliant pantry staple. Buy them tinned in juice (without extra sugar) and they can be on hand to provide a shot of natural sweetness and fibre – and are delicious with almond. The oats bulk this smoothie out to make it a satisfying brekkie on the go.

SERVES 2

450ml very cold semi-skimmed milk
   or unsweetened almond milk
   (roasted, if wished)
130g drained tinned pitted prunes
   (tinned in juice)
40g almond butter
25g porridge oats
ice, to serve (optional)

1 Blend all the ingredients together in a blender or food processor until smooth and thick.

2 Pour into two glasses and enjoy, adding ice, if you like, or take with you in a portable drinks bottle. The smoothie will keep for a few days in the fridge.

CARROT CAKE SMOOTHIE

PER SERVING | **19G** PROTEIN | **5G** FAT | **41G** CARBS

 301 CALS prep 5 MINS

Think ahead for this one and pop a sliced banana in the freezer overnight so it's frozen ready for this delicious breakfast shake the following morning.

SERVES 2

1 frozen sliced banana
2 medium carrots, peeled and roughly chopped
2–3 pitted dates
1/2 tsp ground ginger
40g rolled oats
35g vanilla protein powder
1 tsp ground cinnamon
1/4 tsp ground nutmeg
seeds from 2 cardamom pods
360ml unsweetened almond milk
ice, to serve (optional)

1 Combine all the ingredients except the milk in a blender or food processor and blitz until everything is broken up. Add the milk and blitz again until smooth.

2 Pour into two glasses and enjoy, adding ice, if you like, or take with you in a portable drinks bottle.

BREAKFAST FRUIT JARS

PER SERVING | **2G** PROTEIN | **0G** FAT | **24G** CARBS

 124 CALS prep 10 MINS

We make a batch of these on meal prep day and the jars keep the fruit fresh for up to five days. Just avoid fruit such as banana, which will go brown.

EACH VERSION MAKES 2 X 500ML JARS

Version 1:
150g blueberries
180g tangerine pieces (about 2 tangerines)
150g kiwi fruit chunks (about 2 kiwis)
100g raspberries

Version 2:
180g grapes
150g strawberries
180g tangerine pieces (about 2 tangerines)
100g blueberries

Version 3:
150g blackberries
180g pineapple chunks
180g mango cubes
100g fresh cherries

1 Wash your selected fruit and pat dry with a tea towel. Peel and chop up any fruit that needs slicing.

2 Layer the fruit into two 500ml jars – try and put heavier fruit towards the bottom and the lighter fruits at the top so they don't get squashed. This will limit the amount of water in the bottom of the jars (the bit I like the most in all honesty).

3 Seal the jars with their lids and put in the fridge until ready to serve.

KIWI BANANA SMOOTHIE

PER SERVING | **13G** PROTEIN | **6G** FAT | **60G** CARBS

 360 CALS prep 5 MINS

A thick and creamy smoothie that will keep you going till lunch.

SERVES 2

3 kiwi fruits
2 bananas
a thumb-sized piece of ginger, peeled and roughly chopped
200ml chilled milk (any milk is fine, soy, almond, coconut, etc)
200g chilled low-fat yogurt
4 tbsp porridge oats
1 tsp honey (optional, if you like it that bit sweeter)
ice (optional)

1 Slice the top and bottom from each of the kiwis, stand them on a chopping board, then slice down around the outsides to remove the skins.

2 Peel and roughly chop the bananas, then peel and roughly chop the ginger.

3 Put the fruit and ginger into a blender with all the remaining ingredients and blitz until smooth. You can add some ice to the blender to make it extra thick and cold, if you wish.

4 Pour into two tall glasses and enjoy, or take with you in a portable drinks bottle.

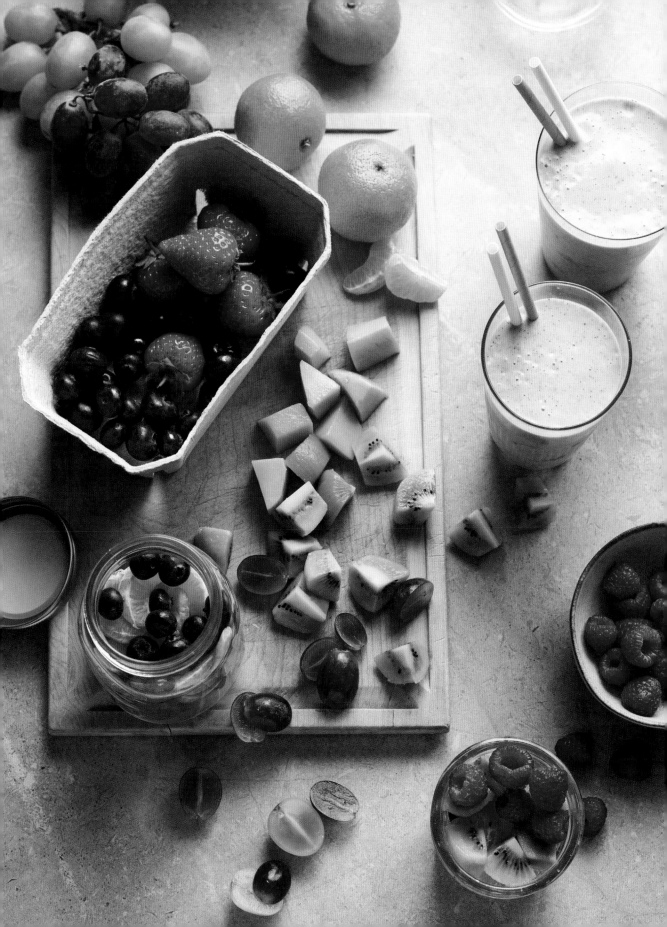

362
CALS

OVERNIGHT BLUEBERRY OATS

PER SERVING | 362 CALS | 21G PROTEIN | 9G FAT | 45G CARBS

prep

5 MINS +
SOAKING

SERVES 2

100g whole rolled oats
300ml unsweetened
   almond milk
1 tbsp chia seeds
2 tbsp protein powder
   (I use vanilla)
2 tsp honey
1/2 tsp vanilla extract
160g fresh or frozen
   blueberries
finely grated zest of 1 lemon

Assemble these the night before so you can take a healthy filling breakfast with you on the go. With zingy lemon and sweet blueberries and vanilla, they taste far more indulgent than they are.

1 Set yourself up with two 400ml glass jars with lids. Into each jar, add half of the ingredients listed opposite. Shake or stir well. Put the lid on the jars and place the oats in the fridge.

2 When you're ready to serve the overnight oats, simply stir the mixture again and serve cold or at room temperature.

tip

You can serve these plain or with additional toppings, such as nut butters, but don't forget to add the extra calories.

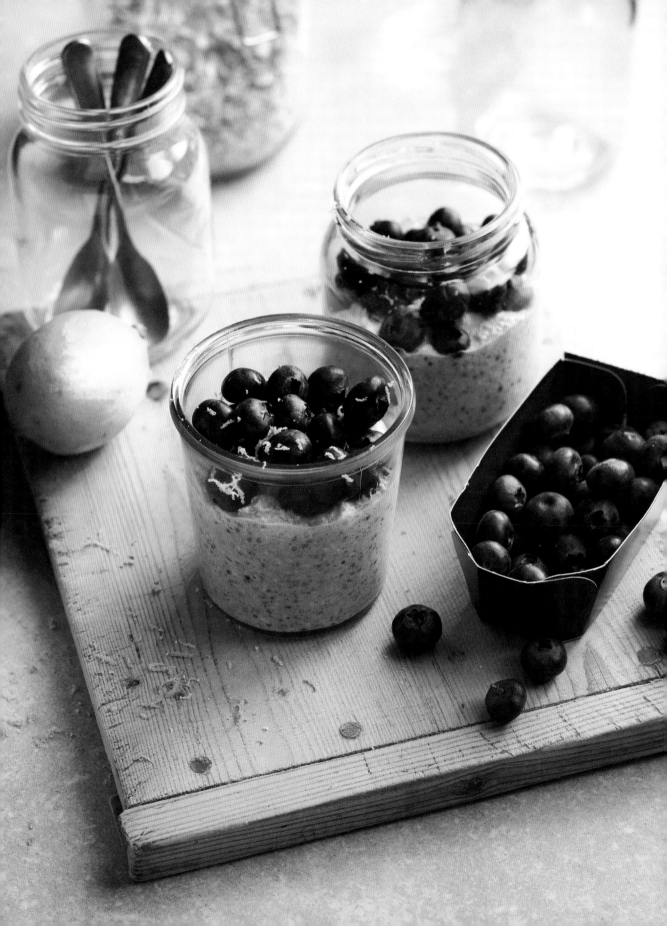

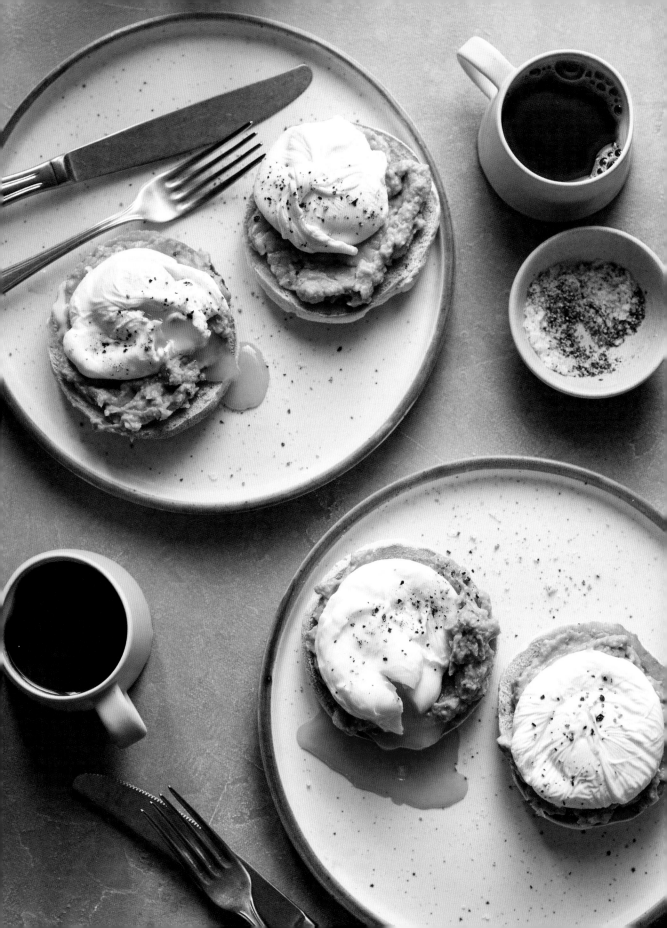

435
CALS

PERFECT POACHED EGGS ON AVOCADO MUFFINS

PER SERVING | **435** CALS | **21G** PROTEIN | **25G** FAT | **29G** CARBS

prep   *cook*

5 MINS   10 MINS

SERVES 2

2 English muffins
1 avocado
juice of ½ lemon
a large pinch of garlic
   granules, to taste
4 ultra-fresh eggs
salt and pepper

tip

If you aren't sure that your eggs are super fresh, add a tablespoon of vinegar (preferably a clear or very pale one, such as white wine vinegar) to the water in the pan, as this will help hold the eggs together.

OK, I admit, it's not really possible to meal prep an egg, but I get asked about my poached eggs so often I had to include them. This is one for if you have a bit more time in the morning. It's so important to use super-fresh eggs for poaching, or they can come apart in the water.

1 Slice the English muffins in half and toast them on both sides.

2 Put the avocado in a bowl and smash it to a chunky purée with a fork. Stir in the lemon juice and garlic granules, then season with salt and pepper and set aside.

3 Fill a large saucepan with water and bring to the boil. Once boiling, turn off the heat completely – we want to poach the eggs not boil them.

4 Crack an egg into a small container such as a ramekin or whatever you have to hand. Stir the water to create a vortex, then add the egg carefully so as not to break the yolk. Quickly crack the other egg into the bowl, then add it to the pan, too.

5 Let the eggs poach in the hot water for 3–5 minutes until the white is solid and opaque and the egg yolk is still soft to the touch. There is no set time here – watch them continuously as judging by eye is the best way to ensure a perfect egg.

6 Once ready, remove the eggs from the water with a slotted spoon and place on kitchen roll. Repeat to cook two more eggs.

7 Meanwhile, spread the smashed avocado over the cut side of each muffin half. Place an egg on top of each muffin half and sprinkle with a little more salt and pepper to serve.

354 CALS

TRIPLE STACK PROTEIN WAFFLES

PER SERVING | **354** CALS | **30G** PROTEIN | **7G** FAT | **41G** CARBS

5 MINS + RESTING   20 MINS   FREEZE

SERVES 4

150g overripe bananas (the browner the banana the better)
120ml skimmed milk
3 eggs
1 tbsp vanilla extract
30g coconut flour
60g plain flour
90g whey protein
½ tsp baking powder
low-calorie cooking oil spray

To serve (per person):
60g berries
1 tbsp plain yogurt
2 tsp honey

These freeze really well, so you could prepare a big batch of them and keep them in the freezer. Reheat in the toaster or the microwave, or enjoy cold.

These actually taste more like cake than a waffle. They are fantastic with ice cream, berries, fat-free yogurt, jam – you name it.

1 In a large bowl, mash up the bananas with a fork. Add the milk, eggs and vanilla and mix until a smooth mixture is formed.

2 Sift in the flours, protein powder and baking powder, then mix thoroughly until you have a nice thick paste-like consistency. Leave the batter to sit for 5–10 minutes.

3 Preheat the waffle maker and spritz with low-calorie oil spray.

4 Divide the mixture into four portions, making three waffles per portion. Add a portion to the waffle maker and cook for about 2–4 minutes until the waffles are set and golden. Repeat to cook the remaining waffles.

5 Serve the waffles topped with berries, yogurt and a little drizzle of honey.

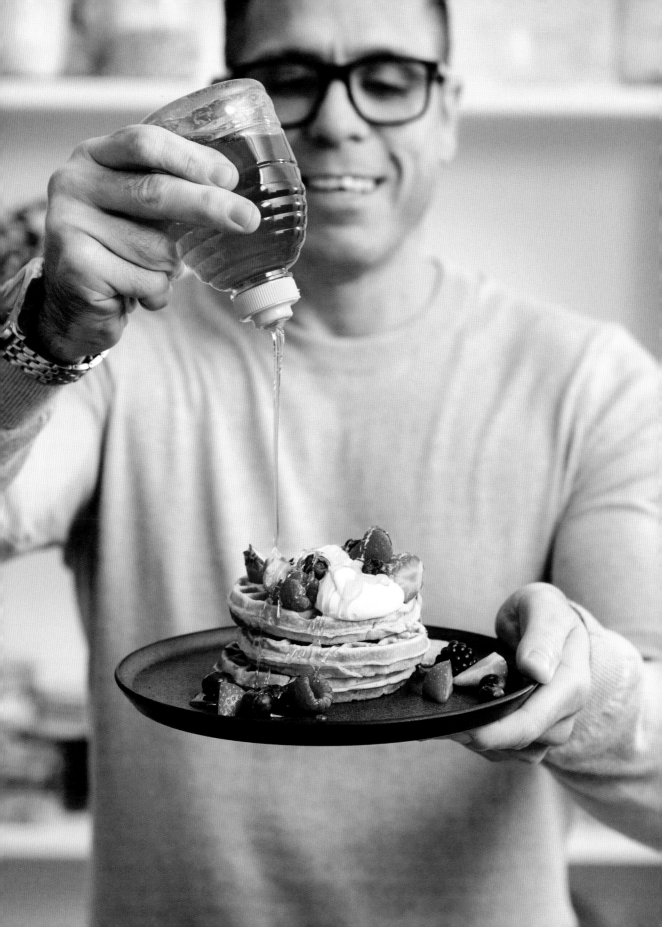

236
CALS

NO-BAKE EASY BREAKFAST BARS

PER BAR | **236** CALS | **6G** PROTEIN | **14G** FAT | **19G** CARBS

prep

15 MINS +
CHILLING

MAKES 12

200g porridge oats
60g whole almonds,
    roughly chopped
40g chocolate chips
40g dried cranberries
½ tsp salt
40g honey
40g coconut oil
130g almond or
    peanut butter

Tired of skipping breakfast because you don't have time? These are great for grabbing on the way out the door in the morning. Or if you aren't a breakfast person, take with you for an energy boost on the go.

1 Line a 20 x 20cm brownie tin with non-stick baking paper.

2 Combine the oats, almonds, chocolate chips, cranberries and salt in a large mixing bowl.

3 Put the honey, coconut oil and nut butter in a small saucepan and heat over low heat until everything is melted and combined. Pour over the oat mixture and mix together really well.

4 Once mixed, transfer to the prepared brownie tin and spread level, then flatten down firmly – a potato masher is useful for this.

5 Cover with cling film and place in the fridge for a few hours to set. Turn out onto a chopping board and cut the block into 12 bars with a sharp knife. Store in an airtight container in the fridge for up to a week.

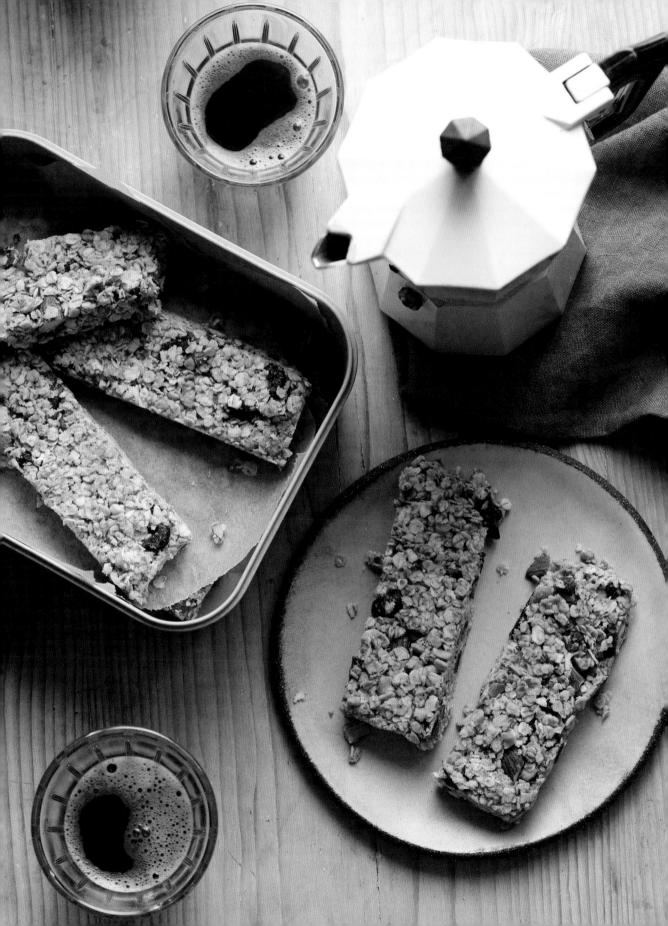

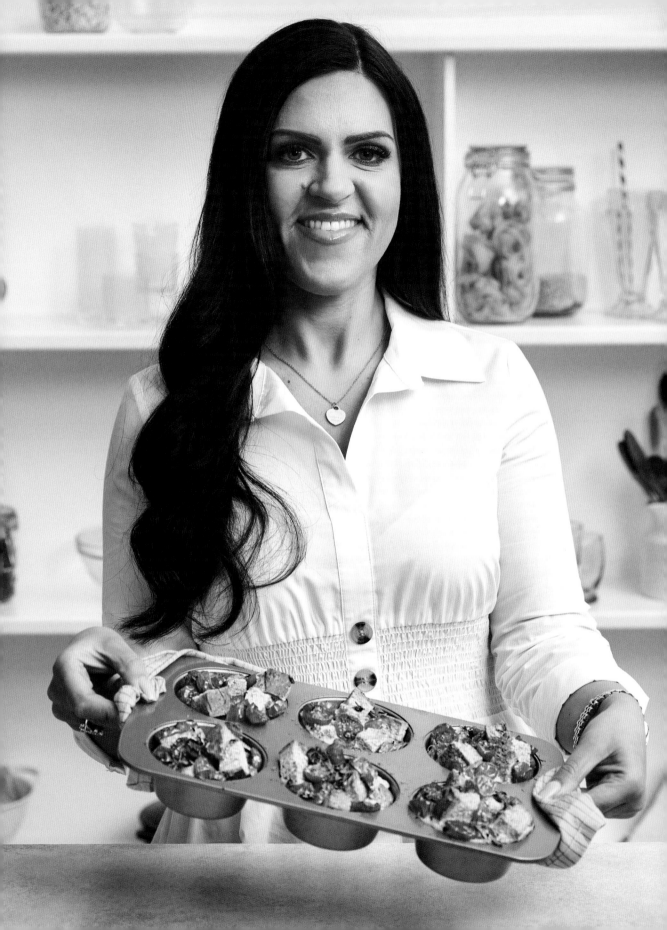

EGG AND TOMATO TOAST CUPS

PER CUP | **212** CALS | **16G** PROTEIN | **10G** FAT | **13G** CARBS

10 MINS   55 MINS   FREEZE

MAKES 6

low-calorie cooking
   oil spray
500g cherry tomatoes
1½ tsp dried thyme
3 x 2cm thick slices
   wholemeal bread
10 large eggs
salt and pepper

If you have bread that's going stale or that needs using up, feel free to use it in this recipe. It works great at bringing the bread back to life.

This is like having egg and tomatoes on toast – only on the go. These are delicious fresh from the oven, or enjoy cold or warmed up in the microwave later on.

1 Preheat the oven to 160°C fan and grease a 6-hole jumbo muffin tin with a few sprays of low-cal spray in each hole.

2 Slice the cherry tomatoes in half and lay them out, cut side up, on a large baking tray. Spritz with a little low-cal spray and sprinkle with the thyme and salt. Roast for 40 minutes until they are like semi-dried sunblush tomatoes.

3 Meanwhile, slice the bread into 2cm chunks. Spread out on another baking tray and again spritz with low-calorie spray. Once the tomatoes have had 25 minutes, pop this tray in the oven under the tomatoes and cook for the remaining 15 minutes the tomatoes have, stirring halfway through, until crisp all over. If the bread is a bit stale, they may only need 10 minutes, so keep an eye on them and remove them from the oven when they are golden and crisp.

4 Once the tomatoes and toast chunks are cooked, whisk together the eggs and season well with salt and pepper. Divide the toast chunks and the tomatoes between the holes of the muffin tray, then pour over the egg, dividing it evenly. Bake for about 15 minutes, or until the eggs are cooked through, and the cups are risen and golden on top. Eat straight away or pop in meal prep containers in the fridge for enjoying later on.

329
CALS

PECAN MAPLE PANCAKES

PER SERVING | **329** CALS | **8G** PROTEIN | **14G** FAT | **41G** CARBS

15 MINS +
RESTING

20 MINS

FREEZE

SERVES 4

50g pecans, plus (optional)
   extra to serve
   (see tip below)
150g plain flour
2 tsp baking powder
1 tsp ground cinnamon
½ tsp ground ginger
½ tsp ground nutmeg
a pinch of salt
1 large egg
110g tinned pumpkin purée
3 tbsp maple syrup, plus
   a drizzle extra to serve
150ml semi-skimmed milk
1 tbsp butter, for cooking

*You can add a few extra
pecans for sprinkling
over the top and an extra
drizzle of maple syrup, if
you like, but don't forget
to add the calories.*

*These pancakes with toasty nuts, spices and sweet pumpkin
are great for a warming start on a cold morning.*

1 Preheat the oven to 180°C fan and tip the pecans onto
a small baking tray. Pop in the oven for about 5 minutes,
or until they have darkened slightly in colour and are
smelling toasty. Set aside to cool a little.

2 Sift the flour and baking powder into a bowl and stir
in the ground spices and salt.

3 In another bowl, beat together the egg, pumpkin purée,
maple syrup and milk. Add the flour mixture and stir
everything together well. Leave to rest for 15 minutes or so.
In the meantime, chop the pecans and add 40g to the batter;
reserve the remaining pecans for sprinkling on the top.

4 Heat the butter in a large non-stick frying pan over medium
heat. Use a ladle to spoon puddles of the batter into the pan,
spacing well apart. Cook for a couple of minutes until you can
see the top is starting to set, then flip the pancakes over and
cook on the other side until firm and golden all over. Repeat
to cook the rest of the batter – you should be able to make
about 12 small pancakes.

5 If serving straight away, drizzle with a little maple and
sprinkle over some of the reserved pecans. If meal prepping,
pop in a container and keep a little syrup in a separate pot
for drizzling over just before eating.

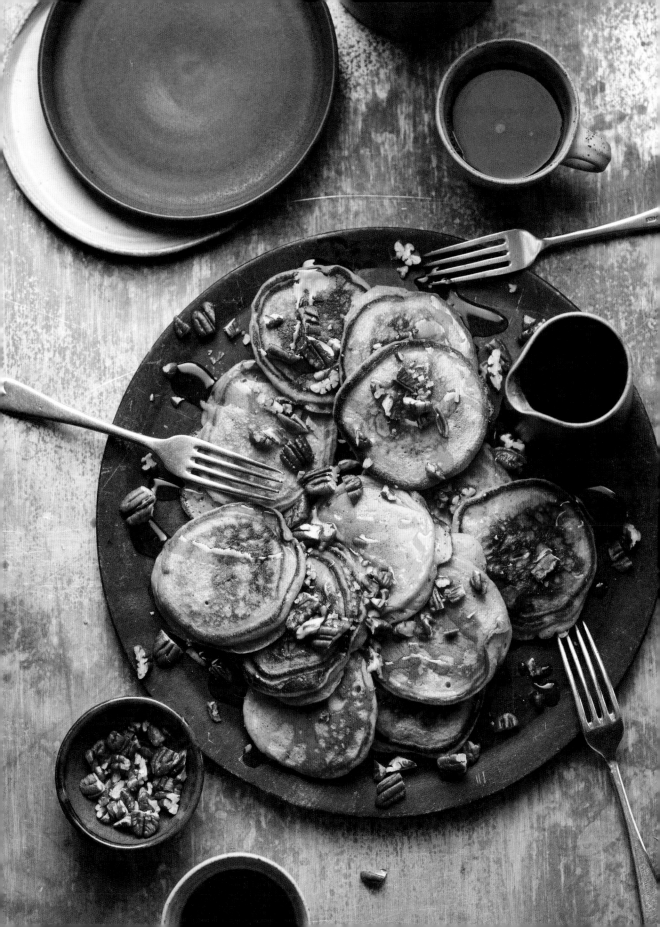

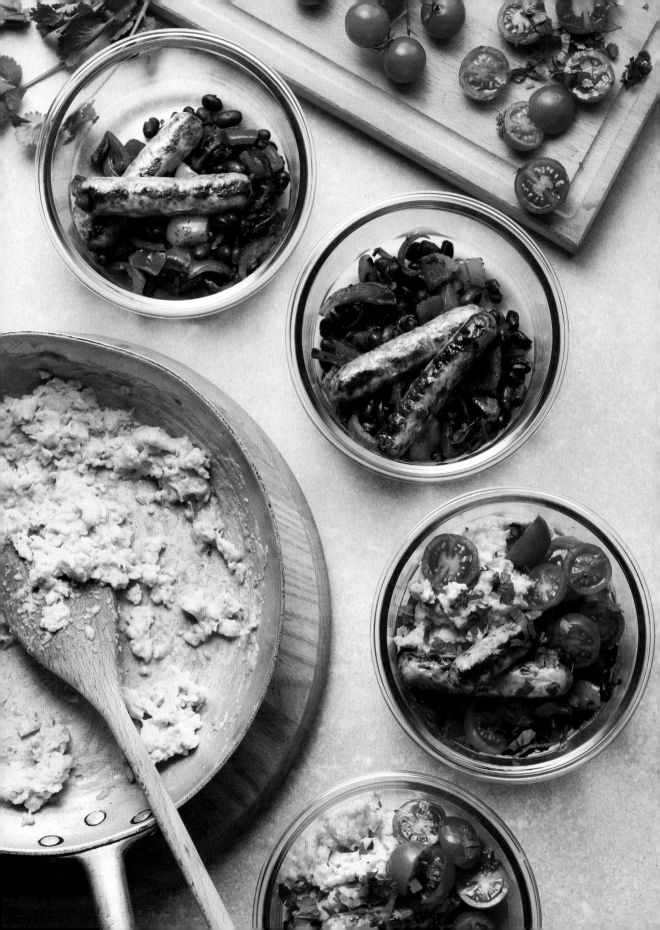

486
CALS

SCRAMBLED EGG AND SAUSAGE BREAKFAST BOWLS

PER SERVING | **486** CALS | **39G** PROTEIN | **23G** FAT | **27G** CARBS

prep   cook
10 MINS   25 MINS

SERVES 4

1 tbsp olive oil
1 red onion, sliced
2 garlic cloves, minced
1 green pepper, chopped
1 yellow pepper, chopped
1 tsp taco seasoning
1 x 400g tin black beans,
    drained
8 low-fat sausages
8 eggs
80g low-fat grated cheese
200g cherry tomatoes,
    halved
salt and pepper
a small bunch of fresh
    coriander or parsley,
    chopped, to garnish

tip

*Check the nutritional info
on packets of sausages as
calories can vary greatly.
Chicken sausages tend
to be lower in calories.*

*A substantial breakfast that can be enjoyed hot or cold.
Cooking the eggs in the same pan as the sausages may
discolour them a little, but it adds tons of extra flavour.*

1 Heat half the oil in a large sauté pan over a medium heat.
Add the onion, garlic and peppers and taco seasoning, then
sauté until softened, about 5–6 minutes. Add the black beans
to the pan, stir well and cook for 1 more minute. Season with
salt and pepper, then scrape the contents of the pan onto
a plate and set aside.

2 Fry the sausages in the same pan until golden brown, about
12–15 minutes, then remove from the pan and allow to cool.

3 In a mixing bowl, whisk together the eggs and cheese
and season with salt and pepper. Heat the remaining oil in
the same pan, still over a medium heat. Add the eggs and
cook, stirring continuously, until scrambled to your liking.

4 Divide the scrambled eggs between four meal prep
containers, then add the sausages and onion and pepper
mixture and top with the cherry tomatoes. Garnish with
chopped fresh herbs. Eat hot or cold.

226
CALS

FRENCH TOAST

PER SERVING | **226** CALS | **11G** PROTEIN | **8G** FAT | **26G** CARBS

10 MINS   20 MINS

SERVES 4

2 eggs
1 tsp vanilla extract
½ tsp ground cinnamon
100ml skimmed milk
4 thick-cut slices bread
low-calorie cooking
   oil spray
4 tbsp Greek yogurt
strawberries and/or
   blueberries
a drizzle of maple syrup
   (optional), to serve

*To make this savoury,
simply omit the vanilla
and cinnamon from the
batter mixture. Prepare
and cook the toast as
in the recipe opposite
and top with bacon, eggs,
tomatoes or ketchup, etc.*

*What I love about this is how adaptable it is – I used to
have this as a savoury meal as a kid, but it can be made
sweet as shown and any fruit can be used. I have this
as a midnight snack too when we have not much food
in and need to go shopping.*

1 In a mixing bowl, beat together the eggs, vanilla and
cinnamon, then stir in the milk. Pour it into a wide shallow
container, such as a baking dish or tray, in which you can
lay out all the bread slices in a single layer (you may need
to use 2 dishes). Lay the bread slices in the mixture and turn
over to coat both sides. Leave the slices in the mixture
until it is all absorbed by the bread.

2 Heat up a non-stick frying pan over a low–medium heat
and spray liberally with cooking oil spray. Add as many slices
as will fit in the pan at a time and cook for 3–4 minutes until
golden brown. It's important not to have the heat too high
or the outside will burn before the middle is warmed through.
Turn over and cook on the other side until golden brown all
over. Remove from the pan and repeat to cook the other slices.

3 Top the toast with a dollop of Greek yogurt and the
berries, and add a drizzle of syrup to serve, if wished.

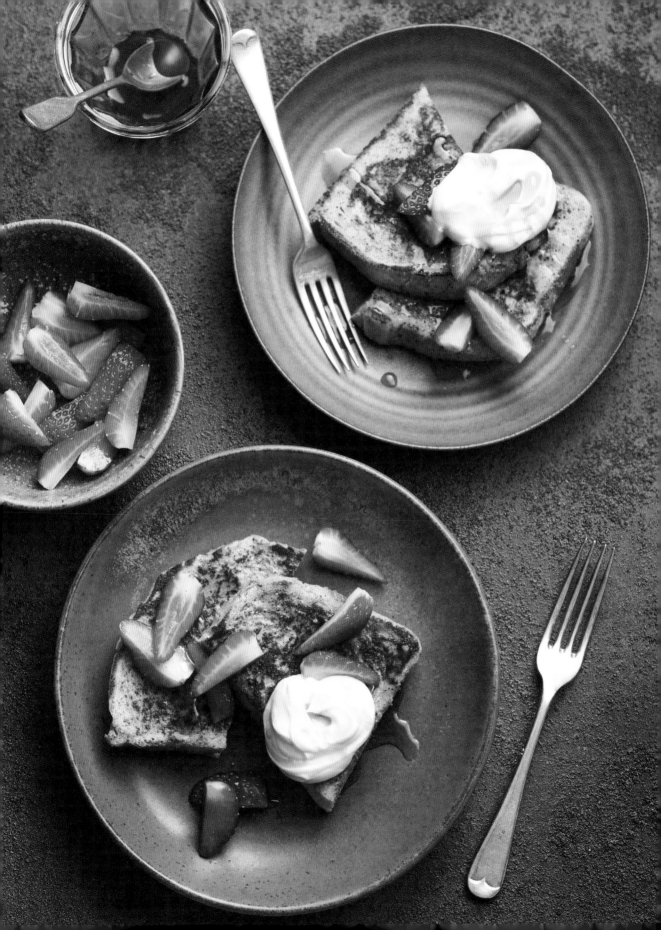

SWEETCORN FRITTERS

PER SERVING | 329 CALS | 14G PROTEIN | 13G FAT | 35G CARBS

prep 10 MINS   cook 15 MINS   FREEZE

SERVES 4 (MAKES 12)

420g tinned, drained
  sweetcorn kernels
6 tbsp plain flour
1 tsp paprika
2 medium eggs
juice of ½ lime
a handful of fresh
  coriander, plus extra
  leaves to serve
½ small onion, finely diced
2 tsp olive oil
salt and pepper

To serve:
4 tbsp low-fat Greek yogurt
1 avocado, peeled, pitted
  and diced (see note
  in method)
sliced rings of red chilli

tip

*You can also use fresh
corn on the cob for an
extra sweet taste and
a lovely crunch.*

*An easy recipe the whole family can enjoy, especially the
kids. Feel free to top with a fried egg for extra calories.*

1 Tip half the drained sweetcorn kernels into a food processor,
setting aside the other half. To the processor, add the flour,
paprika, eggs and lime juice and season with a little salt and
pepper. Blitz until the mixture is almost smooth. Add most of
the coriander and pulse a couple of times until it is roughly
chopped into the batter – you want the flecks of green to
still be visible.

2 Tip the batter into a bowl and stir in the reserved whole
sweetcorn kernels and the finely chopped onion. You should
end up with a thick, chunky batter. Season with salt and pepper.

3 Heat half the oil in a large non-stick frying pan on
medium heat and spoon half of the batter into the pan
to make six circular patties. Fry for 2–3 minutes, until golden
and the fritters have set, then flip over and fry the other
sides for another couple of minutes until golden. Remove
from the pan and repeat to cook the remaining batter
to make 12 fritters in total.

4 Serve 3 fritters per person and top with Greek yogurt,
fresh coriander, avocado dice and chilli. If using as meal prep,
skip this step until serving and keep the toppings stored in
separate little tubs. Halve and quarter the avocado and remove
the pit, keeping the skin on. Squeeze a little lime juice over
it and wrap tightly in cling film to stop it discolouring.
Chop up just before serving.

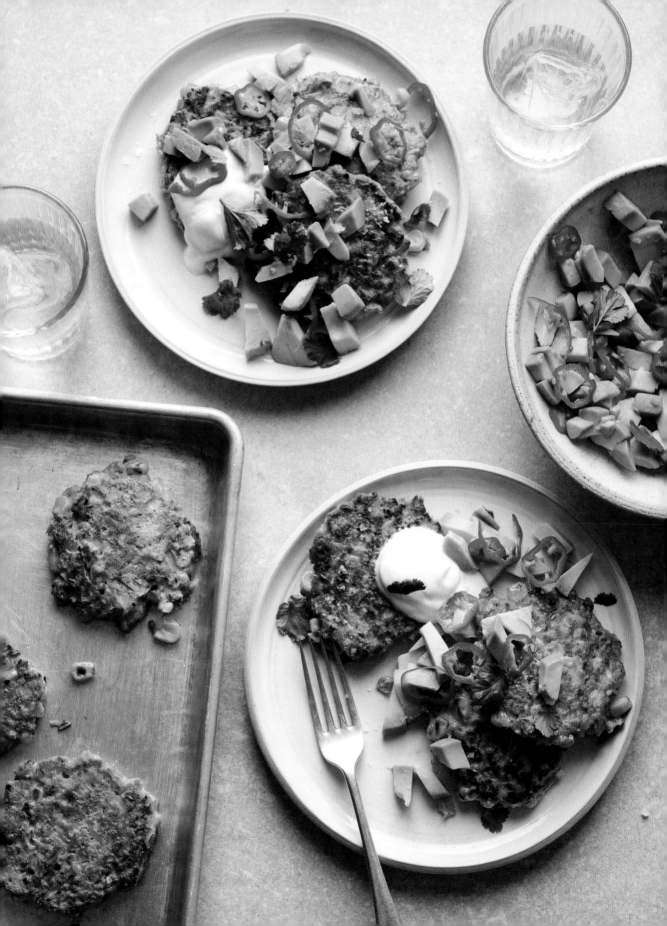

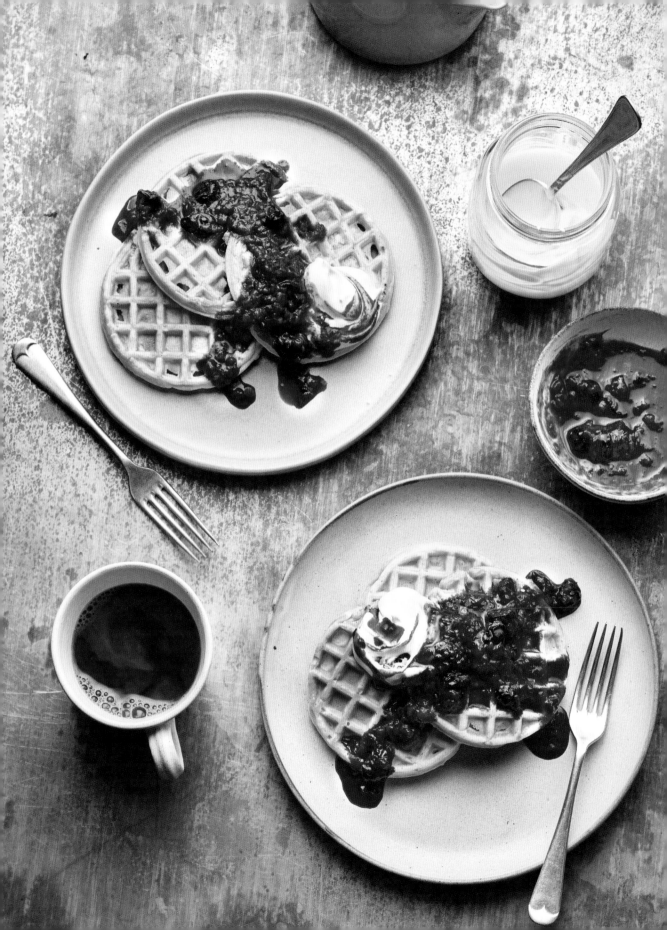

230
CALS

ORANGE BUTTERMILK WAFFLES WITH FROZEN BERRY COMPOTE

PER SERVING | **230** CALS | **12G** PROTEIN | **2G** FAT | **39G** CARBS

10 MINS   15 MINS   FREEZE

SERVES 4

200g buttermilk
1 large egg
1 tsp orange extract
1½ tbsp soft brown sugar
100g plain flour
1 tsp baking powder
½ tsp salt
low-calorie cooking
   oil spray
4 tbsp low-fat Greek
   yogurt, to serve

For the compote:
400g frozen berries
1 tbsp granulated
   sweetener (optional)
1 tsp vanilla extract

These fluffy, fruity waffles make use of any bags of frozen berries you may have in your freezer, and orange and berry always makes a lovely combination. Just chuck in whatever fruit is available.

1 First make the compote. Pop the frozen berries in a saucepan with the sweetener, if using, and vanilla extract. Cook over low–medium heat for about 10 minutes until the berries have broken down into a chunky compote.

2 Meanwhile, whisk together the buttermilk, egg and orange extract until well combined. Sift in the flour, then add the sugar, baking powder and salt and stir everything together.

3 Preheat the waffle maker if you haven't already and spritz it with cooking spray to stop your waffles sticking. Half-fill the machine with batter and close the lid. Cook for 4 minutes or so until the waffles are set and golden, then remove and repeat to cook all the remaining batter. Divide between four plates or meal prep containers. If you are serving straight away, top with a dollop of the compote and a blob of yogurt. If keeping for later, pack the compote and yogurt in small containers to be added just before eating. Reheat the waffles and compote in the microwave and finish with the cold yogurt.

214
CALS

BREAKFAST BRAN MUFFINS

PER MUFFIN | **214 CALS** | **6G PROTEIN** | **4G FAT** | **37G** CARBS (IF USING BRAN FLAKES)

prep
10 MINS

cook
20 MINS

FREEZE

MAKES 12

250g bran cereal
   (any you wish), crushed
300ml skimmed milk
60g soft brown sugar
2 eggs, beaten
1 tsp vanilla extract
40g honey
125g plain flour
2¹/2 tsp baking powder
1 tsp ground cinnamon
¹/2 tsp salt
100g raisins
50g flaked almonds

tip

*Don't have any muffin
cases? No problem.
Use baking paper cut
into 8cm squares and
press into the muffin
trays to create your own.*

*Frank's bran muffins are a low-calorie breakfast idea best
enjoyed with a cup of tea. Why not add one to the kids'
lunch boxes for a morning break snack?*

1 Preheat the oven to 180°C fan and line a 12-hole muffin
tray with non-stick paper cases.

2 Crush the bran cereal in a bowl, then add the milk and
let it sit for 2–3 minutes to soften.

3 Add the brown sugar, eggs, vanilla and honey to the soaked
bran cereal and stir to combine well. Then add the flour, baking
powder, cinnamon and salt and mix in, making sure you don't
overmix. Finally, gently fold in the raisins and flaked almonds.

4 Divide the mixture evenly between the muffin cases and
bake for 15–20 minutes until risen and golden. Enjoy warm
straight from the oven or cold, or flash in the microwave
for a few seconds to reheat later on.

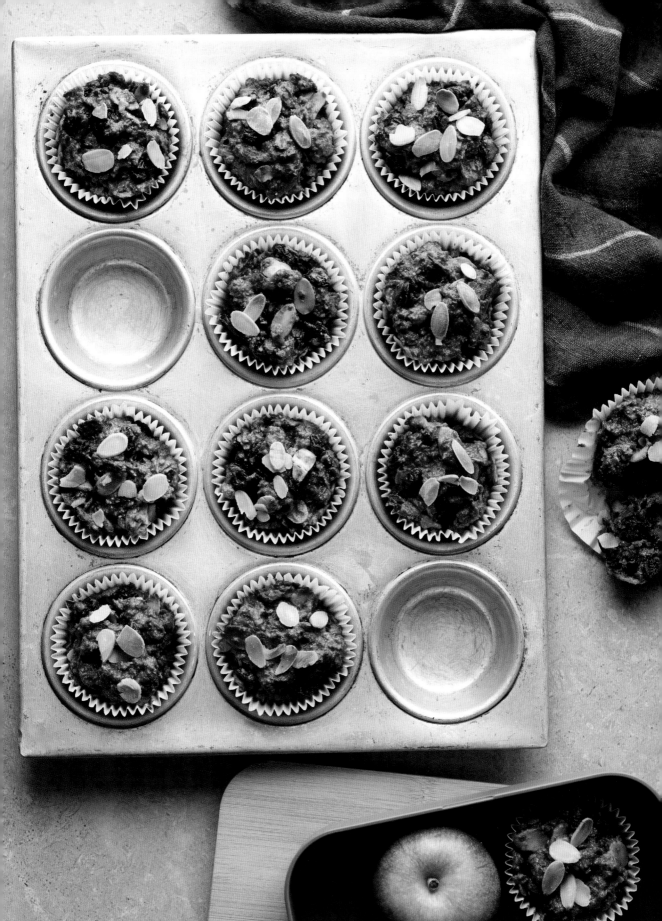

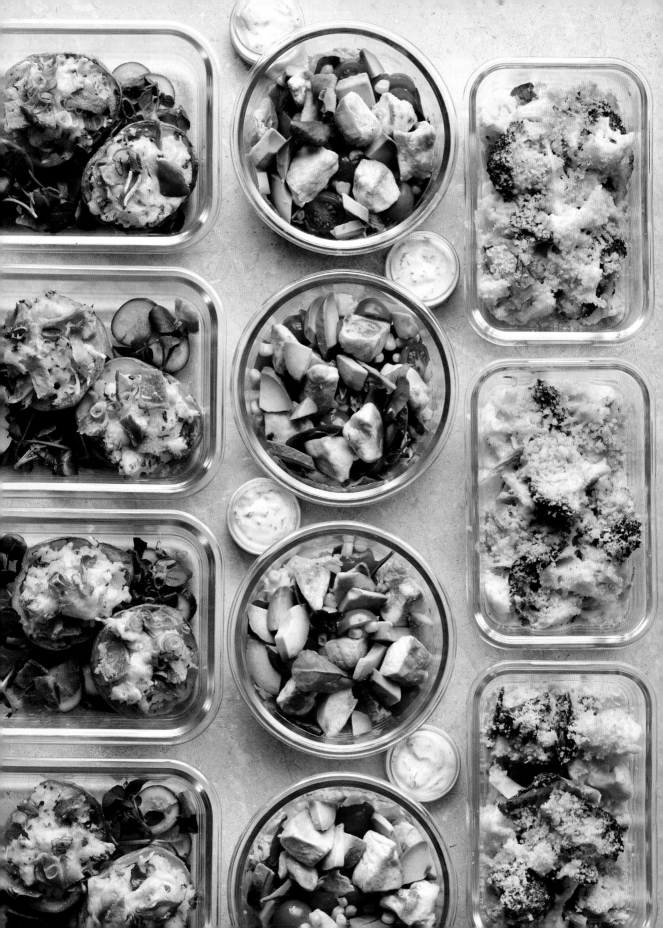

LUNCH

194 CALS

PLUM TOMATO, BASIL AND RED LENTIL SOUP

PER SERVING | **194** CALS | **10G** PROTEIN | **4G** FAT | **28G** CARBS

prep
10 MINS

cook
30 MINS

FREEZE

SERVES 4

1 tbsp olive oil, plus
   extra to drizzle
1 red onion, finely diced
2 large garlic cloves, sliced
1 vegetable stock pot
2 x 400g tins plum
   tomatoes in juice
120g red lentils
1 tsp sugar
1 x 25g pack fresh basil
salt and pepper
fresh bread, to serve

tip

If you like, you can switch the tinned plum tomatoes for fresh ones. Markets often sell tomatoes cheaper later in the day to avoid food waste, so you can get a big bowl of fresh ones for a bargain.

The lentils in this soup help to make it hearty and filling. Serve with an extra generous drizzle of olive oil and more fresh basil leaves to make it feel like you're enjoying this on the Med!

1 Heat the oil in a large saucepan over a low heat and add the onion. Fry gently for 5 minutes until softened, then add the garlic and fry for another 2 minutes.

2 Meanwhile, put the stock pot in a jug and measure in 700ml of boiling water from the kettle. Stir until the stock is dissolved.

3 Add the plum tomatoes to the pan and turn up the heat up to medium. Use a little of the stock to quickly swill out the tomato tins to pick up all the remaining tomato juice, then tip all that water and the remaining stock into the pan. Stir in the sugar and a little salt and pepper and cook for 20 minutes or so until the lentils are tender, stirring occasionally so they don't stick to the bottom of the pan.

4 After this time, turn off the heat and chuck most of the basil into the pan. Blend using a stick blender, or transfer to a blender or food processor and blitz until smooth. This will make quite a thick soup, but if you'd like it runnier, just add more hot water, a little splash at a time, until you get the desired consistency. Check the seasoning and add extra salt and pepper to taste.

5 Either enjoy straight away, topped with the reserved basil leaves and a drizzle of olive oil, with some bread on the side for dipping, or transfer to meal prep containers to be reheated and enjoyed another day.

234
CALS

CURRIED LENTIL SOUP

PER SERVING | **234** CALS | **13G** PROTEIN | **5G** FAT | **32G** CARBS

10 MINS   35 MINS   FREEZE

SERVES 4

1 tbsp olive oil
1 small onion, diced
1 celery stick, diced
1 small carrot, peeled
    and diced
1 garlic clove, crushed
2 tsp mild curry powder
½ tsp ground turmeric
200g red lentils
850ml hot vegetable stock
salt and pepper
a little cream, to serve
chopped fresh coriander,
    to serve

*Leftover coriander? Don't
throw it away; freeze any
leftover fresh herbs to
add to curries or soups
at a later date.*

*Warm, thick and comforting. Serve with one of Frank's
homemade rolls (see page 177) for a seriously satisfying
lunch that's under 500 calories.*

1 Heat the olive oil in a large saucepan over low heat and
gently cook the onion, celery, carrot and garlic for 7–8 minutes
until softening. Add the curry powder and turmeric and cook
for a couple more minutes.

2 Add the lentils, vegetable stock, and increase the heat
to bring to a simmer. Cover with a lid, turn down the heat to
medium–low and simmer for 20–25 minutes until the lentils
are cooked.

3 Use a stick blender to blitz the soup until smooth -
or transfer it to a food processor or blender and blitz.
Season to taste with salt and pepper.

4 Either enjoy straight away, swirled with a little cream
and topped with a few coriander leaves, or transfer to meal
prep containers to be reheated and enjoyed another day.

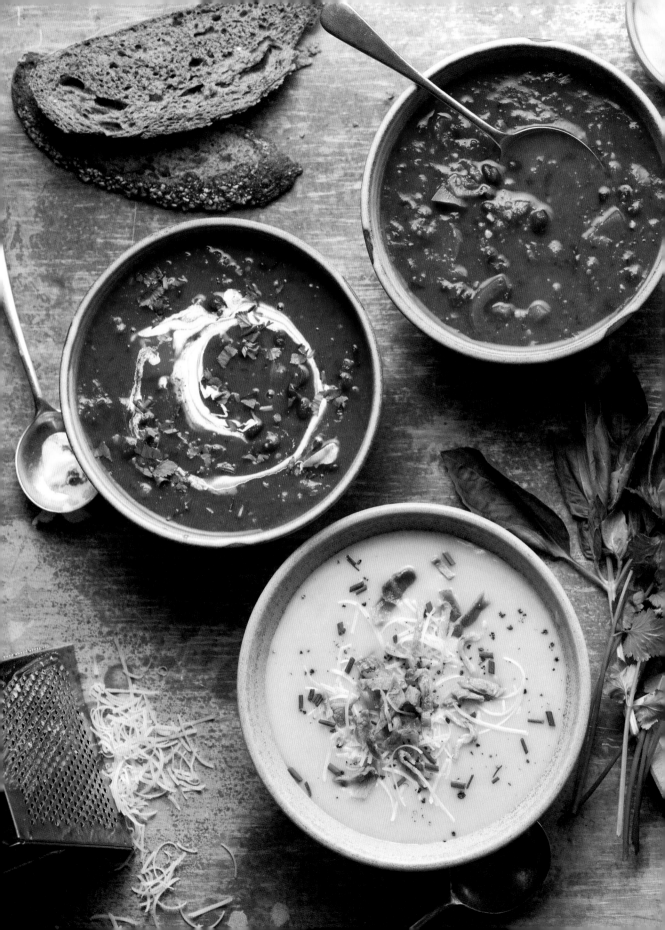

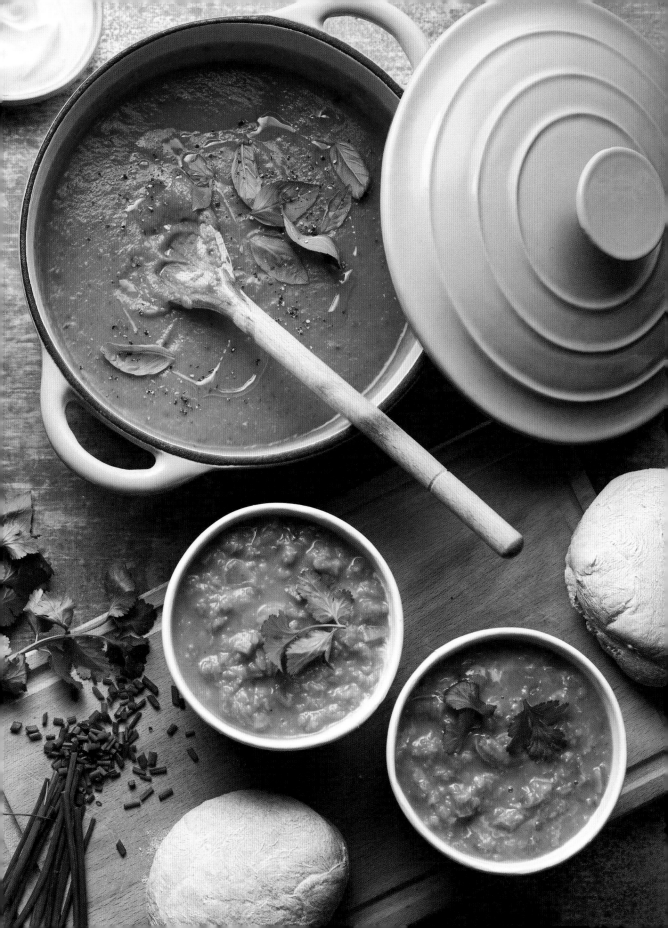

267 CALS

CUBAN BLACK BEAN SOUP

PER SERVING | **267** CALS | **13G** PROTEIN | **8G** FAT | **32G** CARBS

10 MINS   30 MINS   FREEZE

SERVES 4

2 tbsp olive oil
1 onion, diced
1 red pepper,
    deseeded and diced
3 garlic cloves,
    finely chopped
2 tsp ground cumin
1 tsp dried oregano
1 tsp hot smoked paprika
2 x 400g tins black
    beans, drained
1 x 400g tin chopped
    tomatoes
600ml vegetable stock
juice of 1 lime
salt and pepper
soured cream and fresh
    coriander leaves, to serve

This is mildly spiced, hearty and delicious.

1 Heat the oil in a large saucepan and add the onion.
Fry for a good 6–7 minutes until tender. Add the red pepper,
garlic, cumin, oregano and paprika and cook for a couple
more minutes.

2 Add the beans to the pan along with the chopped tomatoes
and vegetable stock. Bring the mixture to a boil, then lower
the heat and simmer for 15–20 minutes, stirring occasionally.

3 Using a stick blender, blitz the soup a little until blended,
but it still has plenty of texture. You can also do this in a food
processor. Add the lime juice and taste and season with salt
and pepper.

4 To serve, divide the soup into bowls or meal prep containers.
Just before serving, add a dollop of soured cream to the top
of each portion, along with a few coriander leaves.

*As this is low in calories,
it is delicious served
with a slice of toasted
sourdough bread.
Don't forget to add
the extra calories.*

290
CALS

SLOW COOKER CHEESY POTATO AND BACON SOUP

PER SERVING | **290** CALS | **16G** PROTEIN | **10G** FAT | **33G** CARBS

prep
10 MINS

cook
3–7
HOURS

FREEZE

SERVES 6

8 slices streaky bacon
1 litre chicken or
    vegetable stock
1kg red potatoes,
    peeled and diced
1 medium onion,
    peeled and diced
120g grated low-fat
    Cheddar cheese
1 tsp salt
1 tsp black pepper
a few snipped fresh
    chives, to serve

tip

You can use bacon with less fat – such as back bacon rashers – for this recipe if you want to reduce the calories further, however the fat in the streaky bacon helps give this recipe huge flavours.

A delicious creamy soup that's filling and just gets better the longer you cook it.

1 Cook the streaky bacon until crisp and golden, either on a baking tray in a hot oven or under the grill, then let cool. (You could fry it, but if you add oil, don't forget to add the extra calories.) Cut up six rashers and add to a slow cooker, then chop the remaining two rashers and set them aside.

2 Add the chicken stock, potatoes and onion to the slow cooker and stir to mix well. Cook on LOW for 5–7 hours or on HIGH for 3–4 hours, or until the potatoes are completely cooked through. (You could also cook this in a saucepan on the hob for about 30 minutes, or until everything is tender).

3 Once the soup has had its time, add 100g of the cheese and stir in until melted. Carefully transfer the contents of the slow cooker to a blender and blitz until smooth. You may have to blend it in two batches – or you could also use a stick blender. Taste and season with salt and plenty of pepper.

4 To serve, divide the soup into bowls or meal prep containers. Just before eating, sprinkle the reserved chopped bacon, remaining shredded cheese, and the chives over the tops of the bowls.

442

CALS

PERI PERI CHICKEN RICE

PER SERVING | **442** CALS | **36G** PROTEIN | **10G** FAT | **50G** CARBS

prep
10 MINS

cook
35 MINS

FREEZE

SERVES 4

2 red peppers, halved
   and deseeded
½ red onion, cut into
   2 wedges
½ lemon
1½ tbsp olive oil
2 garlic cloves
a small handful of
   basil leaves
½ tbsp dried oregano
1 tbsp paprika
1 bird's eye chilli
   (or any red chilli)
4 chicken breasts
180g rice
4 corn on the cobs
salt and pepper
salad leaves, to serve
   (optional)

tip

*Try adding a little low-fat
margarine to the corn on
the cob just before serving,
remembering to add those
calories. It tastes great.*

*A colourful and flavoursome recipe with a little chilli kick
that's great for entertaining guests.*

1 Preheat the oven to 180°C fan.

2 Put the peppers, red onion and lemon half in a baking
dish and drizzle over 1 tbsp of the olive oil. Toss to coat, then
season. Wrap the garlic in foil and pop that in the tray too,
then bake for 25 minutes until the peppers look a little charred.

3 Once cooled, add the peppers and onion to a blender along
with the another 1 tsp olive oil. Squeeze in the juice from the
roasted lemon and squeeze the garlic cloves out of their skins
and add those too. Add the basil, oregano, paprika and chilli,
then blend until a smooth consistency is achieved. Season to
taste with salt and pepper.

4 Butterfly the chicken by slicing the breasts almost in half
down the middle and opening them up. Put the chicken breasts
in a large bowl and cover with the peri peri sauce. Rub the
sauce into the chicken, cover the bowl and leave to marinate
in the fridge for at least 2 hours, or overnight if you can.

5 Heat up a cast iron griddle or non-stick frying pan and drizzle
with a little oil. Cook the chicken breasts for 4–5 minutes on
each side until the chicken is fully cooked – you may have to
do this in two batches, depending on the size of your pan.

6 While the chicken is cooking, cook the rice according to the
packet instructions. In another large saucepan, blanch the corn
cobs for 3–4 minutes, until tender but still with a little crunch.
Once boiled, you can brown the cobs on the griddle, if you like.

7 Serve the chicken with the rice and corn on the cobs, and
a little salad if you like, or pack it into a meal prep container
to enjoy later.

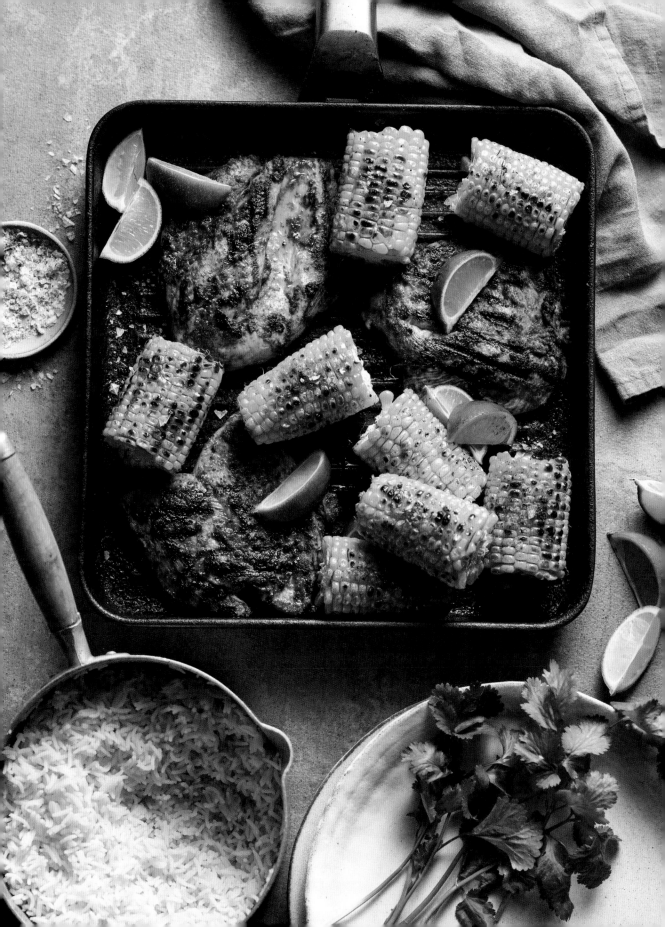

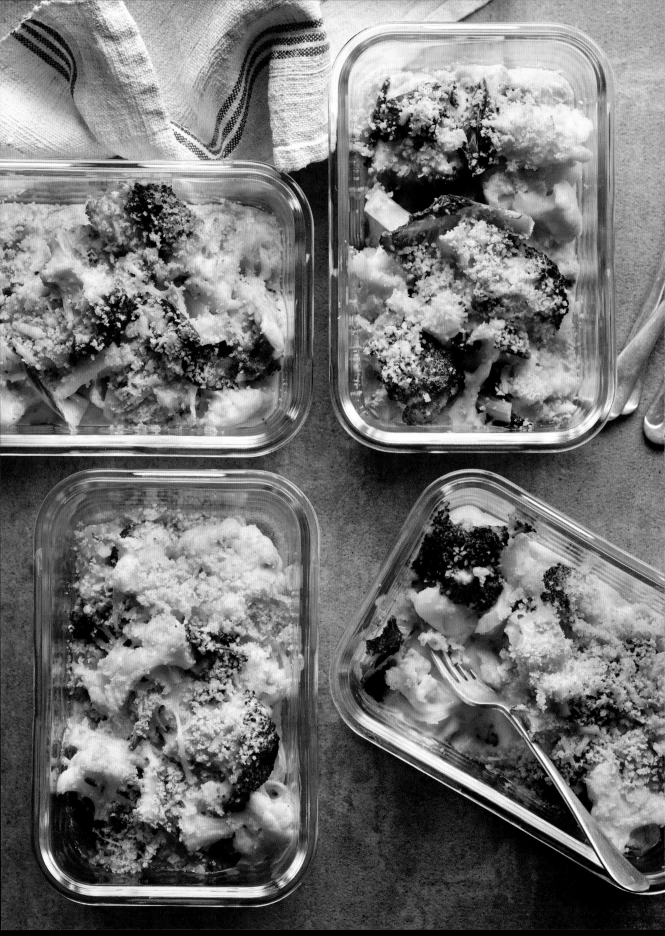

411 CALS

CHEESY BROCCOLI AND CAULIFLOWER BAKE

PER SERVING | **411** CALS | **26G** PROTEIN | **21G** FAT | **26G** CARBS

prep 15 MINS | cook 35 MINS | FREEZE

SERVES 4

600g broccoli florets
600g cauliflower florets
80g light margarine
80g plain flour
800ml semi-skimmed milk
100g low-fat cheese, grated
1 tsp English mustard
    or ½ tsp English
    mustard powder
30g breadcrumbs
low-calorie cooking
    oil spray
salt and pepper

tip

*Don't be afraid to use the
stems of the broccoli and
the cauliflower. There are
lots of fibre and nutrients
here not to be missed –
and less food waste.*

*These make a great veggie meal as they are here.
Or enjoy a dish between two as a side.*

1 Preheat the oven to 180°C fan.

2 Get a large pan of water boiling and blanch all the florets
for 2–3 minutes, until they just begin to soften. Drain them
in a colander and leave them to steam dry in the colander
while you make the sauce.

3 Melt the margarine in a large pan over a medium heat,
then stir in the flour with a balloon whisk. Cook for a minute
before adding a splash of milk. Whisk well to remove any
lumps, then add a little more milk and repeat. Once you have
a smooth runny paste, you can add the remaining milk and
whisk in well. Cook the sauce for at least 5 minutes, until
thickened and the flavour of the flour has been cooked out.

4 Add two thirds of the cheese to the sauce and stir until
smooth. Add the mustard, then taste and season well with
salt and pepper. Once it's to your liking, add the broccoli
and cauliflower florets and stir to coat in the sauce.

5 Divide the mixture evenly between four meal prep dishes
and sprinkle the remaining cheese over the tops. Sprinkle the
dishes with a layer of breadcrumbs and spritz the top of each
one with a little low-calorie cooking spray to help them brown.

6 If you are eating right away, place the dishes in the oven to
bake for 20–25 minutes, until golden brown on top. If you are
keeping them to be used as meal prep, simply seal the dishes
and keep in the fridge until needed.

318 CALS

SPINACH, FETA AND PINE NUT PIES

PER SERVING (2 PIES) | 318 CALS | 10G PROTEIN | 18G FAT | 26G CARBS

prep 30 MINS   cook 45 MINS   FREEZE

MAKES 12 (2 PER SERVING)

50g pine nuts
1 tbsp olive oil
1 onion, finely diced
2 large garlic cloves,
    finely chopped
1 tsp ground allspice
400g spinach leaves
140g cooked rice (from
    a precooked pouch)
160g feta cheese
10g fresh dill,
    roughly chopped
30g butter, melted
6 large rectangular
    sheets filo pastry
salt and pepper

1 Preheat the oven to 180°C fan. Tip the pine nuts onto a baking tray and toast them for 4-5 minutes until golden. Set aside.

2 Heat the oil in a large sauté pan and add the onion. Cook for 7-8 minutes until softened. Add the garlic and allspice and cook for another couple of minutes, then add half of the spinach and pop the lid on. Let it wilt down for a few minutes until there is enough space in the pan to add the remaining spinach. Add the rest and pop the lid on again and cook until it is all wilted. Crumble the rice into the pan and stir in, then stir in the feta, dill and the toasted pine nuts. Season to taste.

3 Brush the holes of a 12-hole muffin tin with the melted butter. Lay out a sheet of filo and slice it widthways into three even strips. Cut each of these in half so you get six squares. Use a square of pastry to line each of the first six holes in the muffin tin, lining the bases and sides and leaving the top overhanging. Pick alternate holes in the tray that are separated from each other so that you don't get confused with the layers of filo! Brush the insides of each filo cup with a little butter. Repeat to add a second square of filo to each cup, rotating the squares so the points come out at different angles and brush again with butter. Then add a third and final square to each cup.

4 Divide half of the filling between the six cups, pushing it down firmly so it all fits snugly. Fold over the overhanging filo, brushing again between each layer as you fold them back in to cover the tops of the pies. Brush the tops of the pies with a little more butter. Repeat to fill and seal the remaining six pies.

5 Bake the pies for about 30 minutes, until crisp and golden. Carefully remove them from the tin whilst still hot or they will steam in the holes and become a little soggy. Enjoy hot or cold. Reheat in a warm oven so the pastry crisps up again.

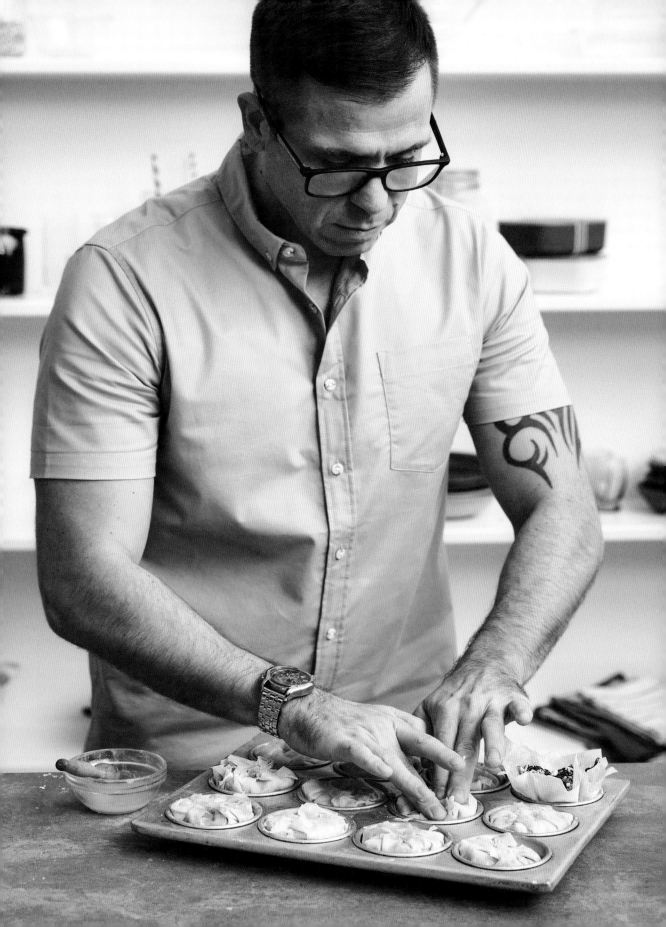

428
CALS

QUICK COCONUT DAHL

PER SERVING | **428** CALS | **17G** PROTEIN | **22G** FAT | **39G** CARBS

PREP 10 MINS | COOK 30 MINS | FREEZE

SERVES 4

1 tsp coriander seeds
½ tsp cumin seeds
½ tsp mustard seeds
1 tbsp coconut oil
1 onion, finely diced
2 large garlic cloves
1 large green chilli,
    finely diced (deseeded
    if you don't want heat)
3cm piece of ginger,
    peeled and grated
1 vegetable stock pot
    or cube
250g red lentils
1 x 400g tin coconut milk
juice of 1 lime
a large handful of
    fresh coriander,
    roughly chopped
salt

Fresh chilli, coriander, lime and coconut give this dahl a south east Asian twist. The red lentils are quick to cook, meaning this one can be knocked up in no time and reheats well in the microwave. Not much to look at, but pretty tasty! Delicious on its own, or serve over rice or with naan if you're feeling particularly hungry.

1 Heat a large saucepan over low–medium heat and add the spice seeds. Toast for a couple of minutes until smelling good, then add the coconut oil and the onion. Cook the onion for a good 6–7 minutes, until tender, then add the garlic, chilli and ginger and cook for a further 1 minute.

2 Dissolve the stock pot in 600ml boiling water from the kettle and add it to the pan along with the lentils and coconut milk. Cook for 15–20 minutes until the lentils are tender, stirring very frequently as the lentils have a habit of sticking to the bottom of the pan. If it is becoming too dry, add a splash more hot water. Once the lentils are cooked, season to taste with salt and stir in the lime juice and most of the coriander.

3 Serve sprinkled with the remaining coriander, or pack into meal prep dishes to be reheated in the microwave another day.

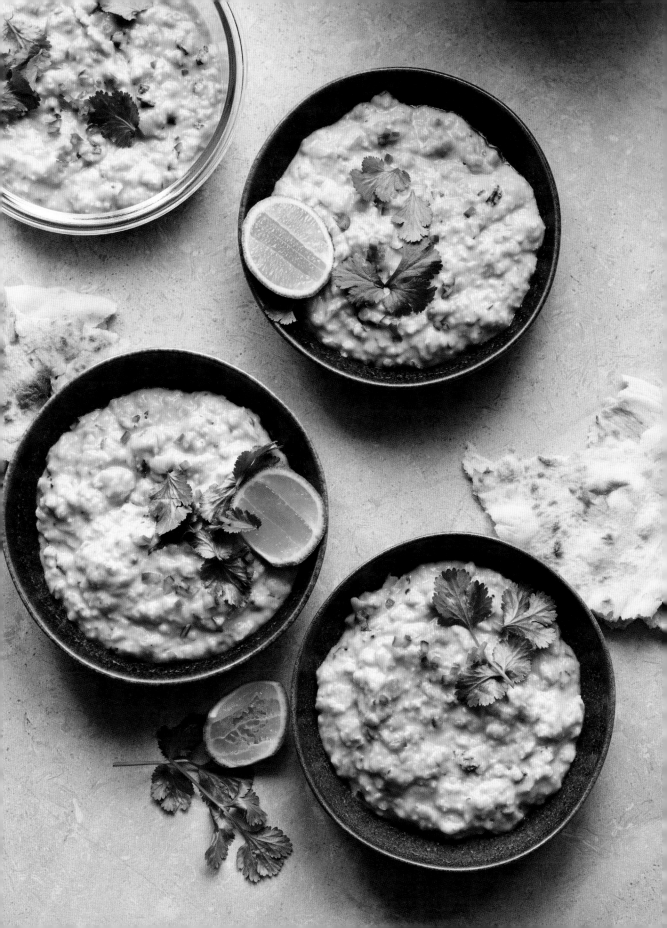

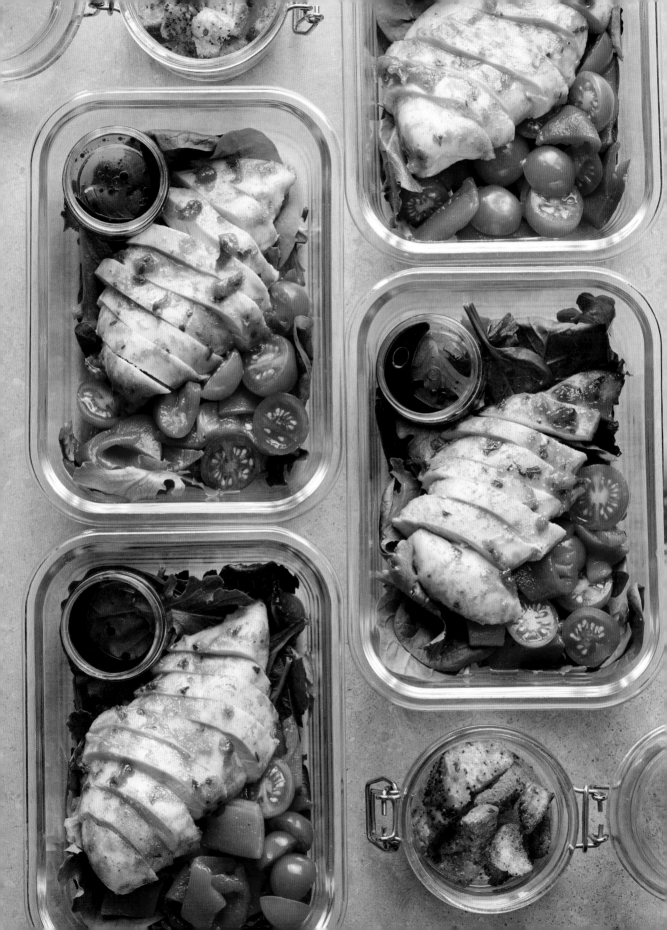

SWEET AND SPICY CHICKEN SALAD

PER SERVING | **285** CALS | **31G** PROTEIN | **8G** FAT | **22G** CARBS

15 MINS   30 MINS   FREEZE

SERVES 4

For the chicken:
zest and juice of 1 lime
4 tbsp apricot jam
1 garlic and herb stock cube
1 tsp cayenne pepper
1 tsp paprika
4 chicken breasts
salt and pepper

For the salad:
2 thick slices slightly
  stale granary bread,
  cut into large dice
a large pinch of paprika
2 tsp balsamic vinegar
60g salad leaves
200g grilled peppers in oil,
  well drained and sliced,
  plus oil from the jar
  (see method)
200g cherry tomatoes,
  halved

*If freezing and reheating,
make sure you don't
reheat the chicken for
too long as this can
make it dry.*

A lower carb meal that's great for getting that extra protein into your daily intake.

1 Preheat the oven to 180°C fan.

2 Mix together the lime zest and juice and apricot jam in a small jar or bowl, then crumble in the stock cube. Add the spices and stir to combine very well.

3 Line an ovenproof dish with kitchen foil. Add the chicken breasts and smother in the jam glaze. Cover with another piece of foil and cook for 15 minutes, then uncover and baste. Cook for a further 10 minutes, uncovered, then baste again. Return the chicken to the oven for a final 5 minutes until golden and cooked through.

4 While the chicken cooks, make the salad. Drizzle the chunks of bread with 2 tsp oil from the pepper jar and toss to coat. Sprinkle with the paprika and salt and bake in the oven with the chicken for about 10 minutes, or until golden add over.

5 Make a dressing by combining another 1 tbsp pepper oil with the balsamic vinegar and seasoning well.

6 Scatter the salad leaves over a plate or into meal prep containers. Add the peppers and tomatoes. Slice the cooked chicken and lay it on top of the leaves and finish with the croutons and a drizzle of dressing. If making this as meal prep, put the croutons and dressing in small containers to add just before eating.

499
CALS

PESTO PASTA BOWLS

PER SERVING | **499** CALS | **17G** PROTEIN | **22G** FAT | **57G** CARBS

prep · cook · FREEZE
10 MINS · 15 MINS · FREEZE

SERVES 4

300g penne pasta
200g cherry tomatoes
   or sundried tomatoes
90g mozzarella pearls

For the pesto:
20g pine nuts
50g fresh basil, plus a few
   small leaves to garnish
20g Parmesan cheese,
   grated
2 garlic cloves
60ml extra virgin olive oil
salt and pepper

*Pesto freezes really well,
so if you are blitzing up a
batch for the pesto pasta,
you could double it and
pop half in the freezer for
a meal prep another day.*

*This is one of my first ever recipes that I still use and
enjoy today as part of my weekly meal prep.*

1 First, put a large saucepan of salted water on to boil
(speed this up by using hot water from the kettle), and
cook the pasta according to the packet instructions.

2 Meanwhile, make the pesto. Toast the pine nuts in a dry
frying pan, stirring constantly, until they're golden brown.
Add to a food blender along with the basil, Parmesan cheese
and garlic cloves and blitz until everything is well chopped.
With the motor still running, trickle in the extra virgin olive
oil and blend until it's a smooth consistency. Season to
taste with salt and pepper.

3 Once the pasta is cooked, drain it in a colander and run
under cold water until the pasta is cold. Return the pasta
to the pan and add the pesto and chopped tomatoes
(or sundried tomatoes) and mix.

4 Divide the pasta between four meal prep containers,
top each with a few mozzarella pearls and garnish with
fresh basil leaves. Store in the fridge and enjoy either
hot or cold.

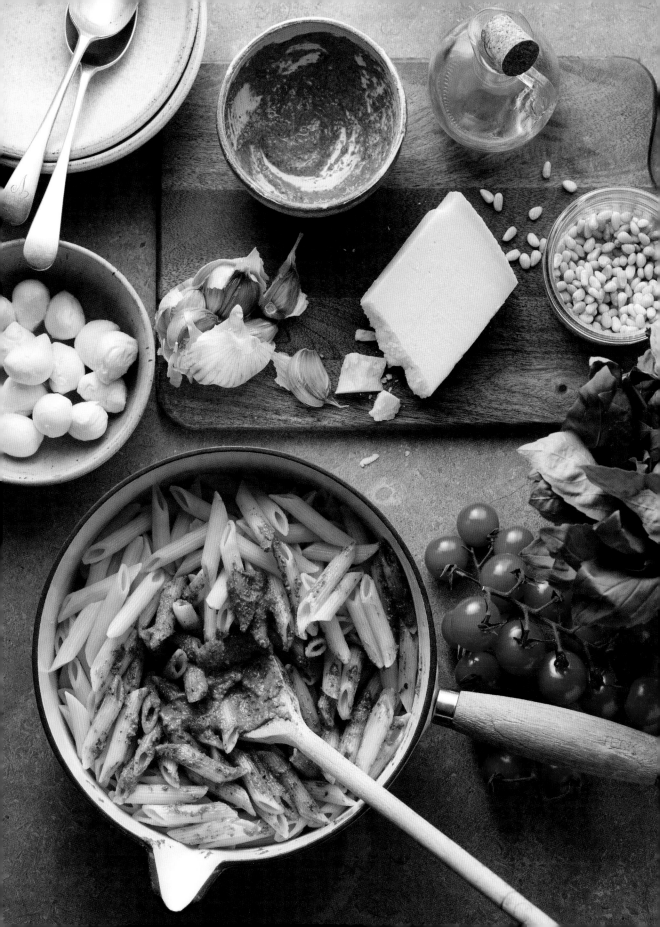

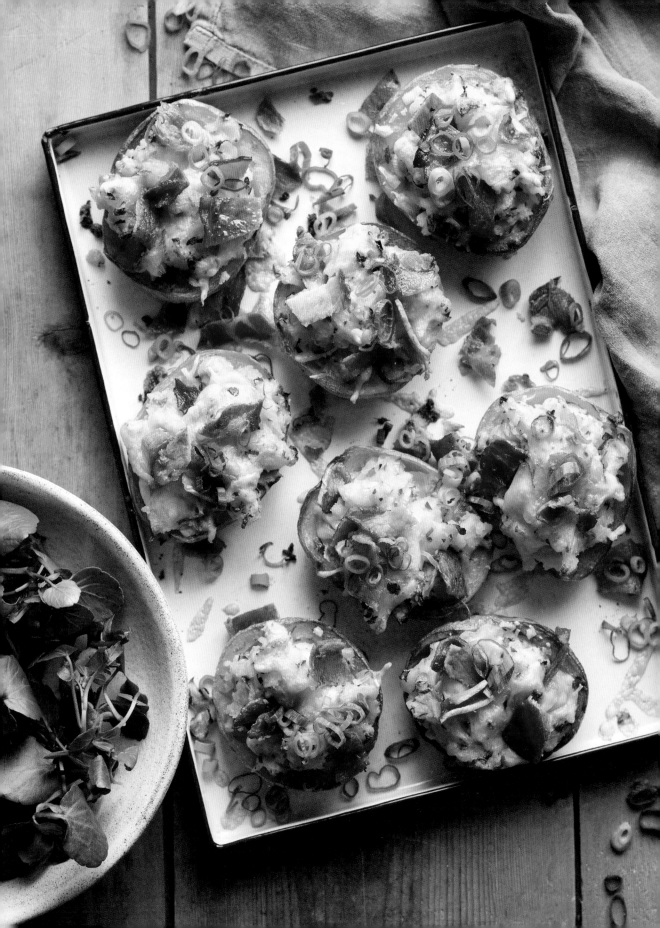

TWICE-BAKED CHEESY POTATOES

PER SERVING | **448** CALS | **19G** PROTEIN | **15G** FAT | **57G** CARBS

prep 15 MINS   **cook** 1 HOUR 30 MINS   **FREEZE**

SERVES 4

4 medium baking potatoes, about 300g each (I like to use Cyprus or Vivaldi)
low-calorie cooking oil spray
2 tsp garlic salt
2 tbsp butter, softened
a small bunch of fresh flatleaf parsley, chopped
6 spring onions, finely sliced and whites and greens kept separate
120g low-fat Cheddar cheese, grated
4 slices back bacon
salt and pepper
salad, to serve

What a way to transform a boring old spud!

1 Preheat the oven to 180°C fan.

2 Wash your potatoes and poke holes in them with a fork. Bake the potatoes for 1 hour, or until crisp on the outside and soft on the inside; you don't want hard potatoes. When the potatoes are cooked, remove them from the oven and cut them in half lengthwise. Scoop out the insides of the potatoes and place the flesh in a bowl, leaving roughly 5mm of the potato on the skins. Increase the oven temperature to 200°C fan.

3 Flip the potato skins over so the skin side is on top and place on a baking tray. Spray with low-calorie cooking spray and sprinkle with the garlic salt. Return the skins to the oven for about 15 minutes to crisp up.

4 While the potato skins are back in the oven, mash the warm potato flesh with a fork. Add the soft butter, parsley, spring onion whites and half the grated cheese and mix well. Season the mixture with salt and pepper to taste.

5 Lay the bacon rashers out on a baking tray. Remove the potato skins from the oven and pop the bacon tray in on the top shelf to cook.

6 Spoon the mixture back into the potato skins and sprinkle the remaining cheese over the tops. If you plan to eat them immediately, place the filled skins back in the oven to cook for 10–12 minutes until the cheese is melted and turning golden on top. If you are meal prepping this, pop them in a container and keep them in the fridge ready to put in the oven later.

7 Once the bacon is cooked and crisp and the tops of the potatoes are golden, serve the skins topped with chopped bacon and the spring onion greens.

250
CALS

CHICKPEA AND FETA SALAD

PER SERVING | **250** CALS | **11G** PROTEIN | **14G** FAT | **17G** CARBS

prep

15 MINS

SERVES 4

For the salad:
1 x 400g tin chickpeas,
   rinsed and drained
1 orange or yellow pepper,
   deseeded and chopped
1 red pepper, deseeded
   and chopped
1 small red onion,
   finely chopped
½ cucumber, diced
200g cherry tomatoes,
   quartered
a handful of fresh
   flatleaf parsley
120g feta cheese, crumbled

For the salad dressing:
1 garlic clove, minced
½ tsp Dijon mustard
2 tbsp extra virgin olive oil
1½ tbsp apple cider vinegar
1 tsp dried oregano
salt and pepper

A colourful and vibrant meal prep that makes you feel healthy. Better than anything you can buy ready-made in a shop.

1 Put the drained chickpeas in a large bowl and add in all of your chopped veggies. Finely chop the parsley and add to the bowl, giving it a mix.

2 Add all the ingredients for the salad dressing to a glass mason jar and shake. Pour over the salad. If making for meal prep, keep the dressing separate.

3 Sprinkle over the feta cheese and serve.

tip

This is delicious with crispy bacon bits sprinkled over the top, but don't forget to add the calories.

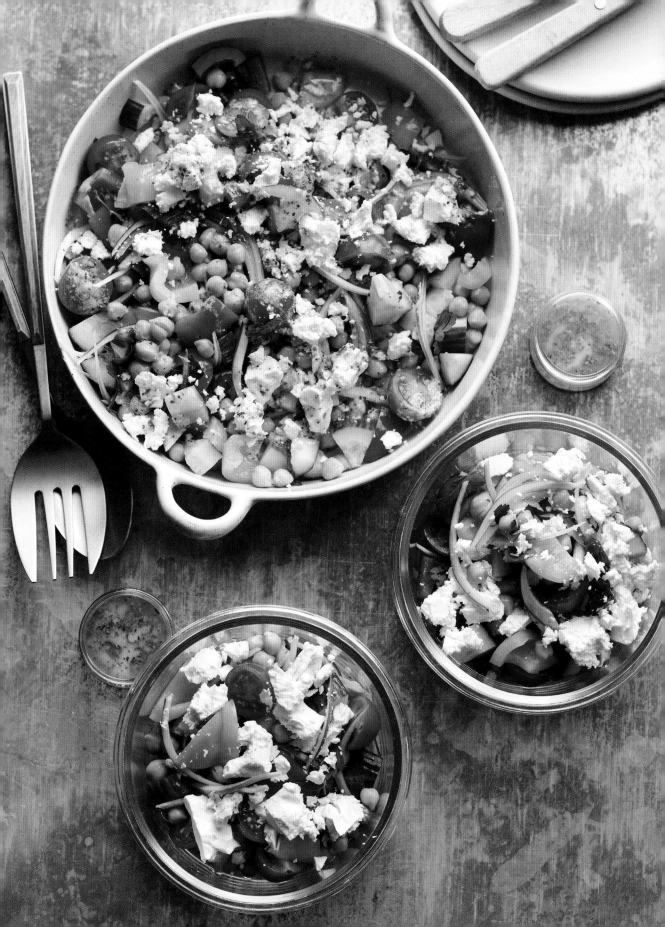

479
CALS

SMOKED MACKEREL AND PINK SLAW WRAP

PER SERVING | **479** CALS | **30G** PROTEIN | **27G** FAT | **27G** CARBS

prep

15 MINS

SERVES 4

4 small smoked
   mackerel fillets
4 wholemeal wraps

For the slaw:
¼ small red cabbage,
   shredded
½ red onion, finely sliced
50g pickled gherkins,
   finely diced
1 eating apple, cored and
   sliced into matchsticks
   (leave the skin on)
150g low-fat Greek yogurt
½ pack fresh dill (15g),
   roughly chopped
juice of ½ lemon
salt and pepper

*Crisp, sweet slaw is great with rich smoked mackerel.
Pile it all into a wholemeal wrap for a satisfying lunch.*

1 To make the slaw, simply combine all the ingredients
in a large bowl. Taste and season with salt and pepper.

2 Divide the slaw between four meal prep containers.
Add a mackerel fillet to each container, roughly flaking
it as you go. Store in the fridge.

3 To serve, give the contents of the container a good
stir, then pile it into a wholemeal wrap and enjoy.

tip

*Heat up your wraps on a
naked flame on a gas hob
for a few seconds either
side – this adds colour
and extra flavour.*

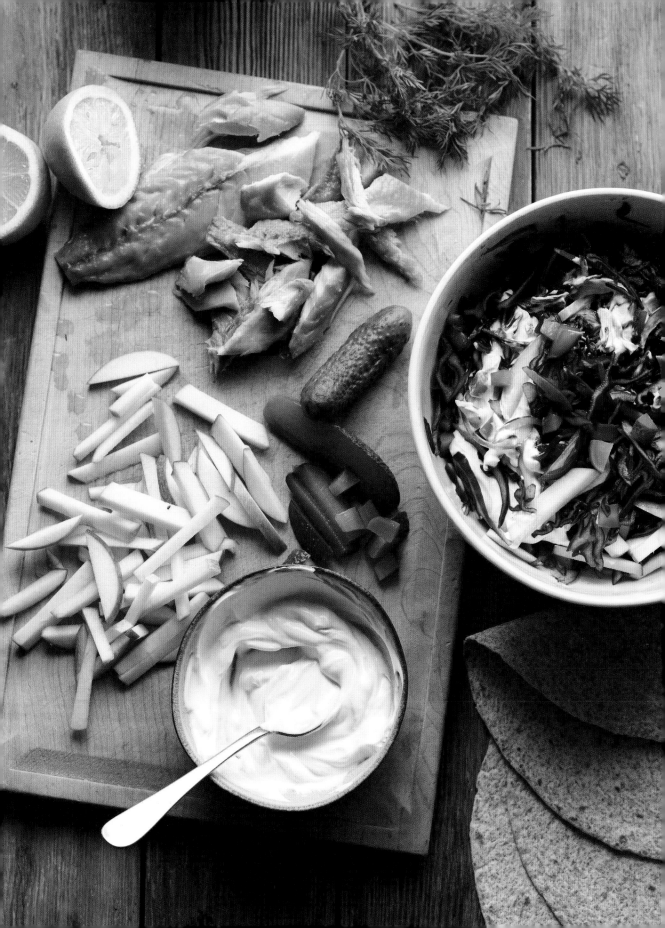

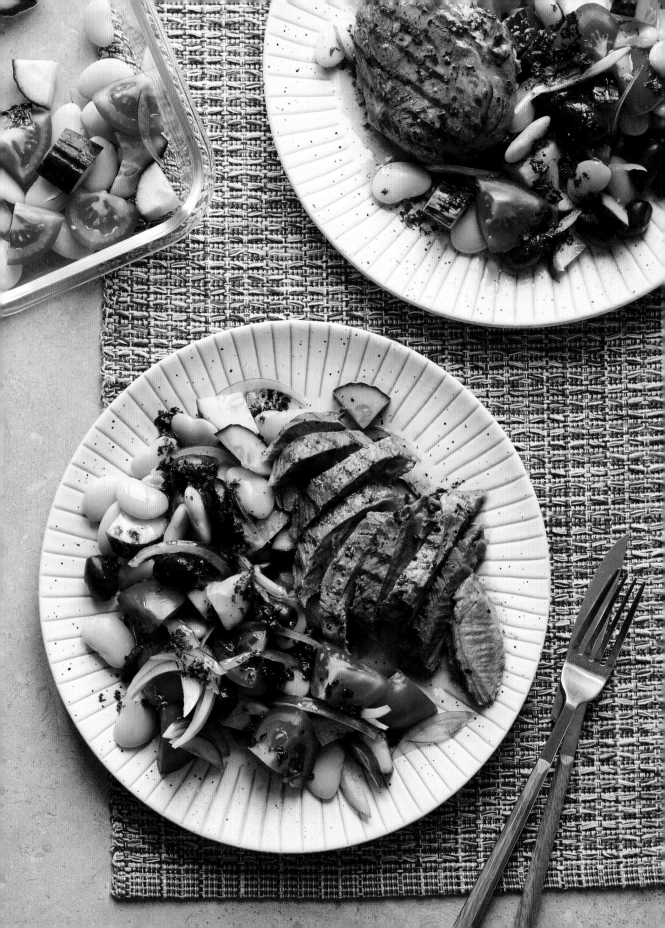

446 CALS

LAMB STEAKS WITH GREEK BUTTERBEAN SALAD

PER SERVING | **446** CALS | **22G** PROTEIN | **28G** FAT | **23G** CARBS

prep 15 MINS   cook 5 MINS

SERVES 4

1 cucumber
6 medium tomatoes
1 small red onion,
    very finely sliced
2 x 400g tins butter beans,
    drained and rinsed
140g pitted black or
    Kalamata olives
4 lamb steaks

For the dressing:
1 large garlic clove
5 tbsp olive oil, plus
    a drizzle for the lamb
juice of 1 lemon
3 tsp dried oregano
1½ tsp dried mint
salt and pepper

This is light and fresh and makes a great dinner or lunch on a summer's day. The beans make it feel substantial and satisfying.

1 Start by making the dressing. Bruise the garlic clove by crushing it slightly with the side of a knife, so that it is flattened and oozing juice, but still in one piece. Pop it into a jug or small bowl and add all the remaining dressing ingredients. Season well with salt and pepper, give it a good stir and set aside.

2 Chop the cucumber into thick slices, then each of these into quarters. Chop the tomatoes in half, then into wedges and halve these, and finely slice the red onion. Tip all the salad veg into a large serving bowl and add the olives and butter beans. Drizzle over the dressing and toss everything together.

3 Drizzle the lamb steaks with a little oil and season well with salt and pepper. Preheat a griddle pan over a high heat until very hot, then lay the lamb steaks on and cook quickly until browned on the outside but still pink in the middle – about 2 minutes on each side should do the trick, depending on how thick your steaks are.

4 Serve the lamb steaks with the Greek salad.

495
CALS

A SIMPLE SALMON SANDWICH

PER SERVING | **495** CALS | **30G** PROTEIN | **25G** FAT | **34G** CARBS

prep
5 MINS

SERVES 2

4 slices of wholemeal bread
a scraping of low-fat
  sunflower spread
1 x 213g tin of boneless wild
  red salmon, drained
2 tbsp low-fat mayonnaise
½ celery stick, finely sliced
¼ red onion, finely sliced
1 tbsp chopped fresh dill
1 tsp Dijon mustard
  (optional)
20g watercress
  or rocket leaves
salt and pepper

A classic, flavour-packed sarnie to take to work, perhaps with some carrot and celery batons or fruit on the side. I will sometimes toast the bread for added colour and crunch.

1 Spread each slice of bread with low-fat spread.

2 In a bowl, mix together the salmon, mayonnaise, celery, red onion and dill and mustard, if using, and season with salt and pepper.

3 Divide the salmon filling between two slices of the bread and top with the salad leaves. Pop the other bread slices on top and slice into halves to serve.

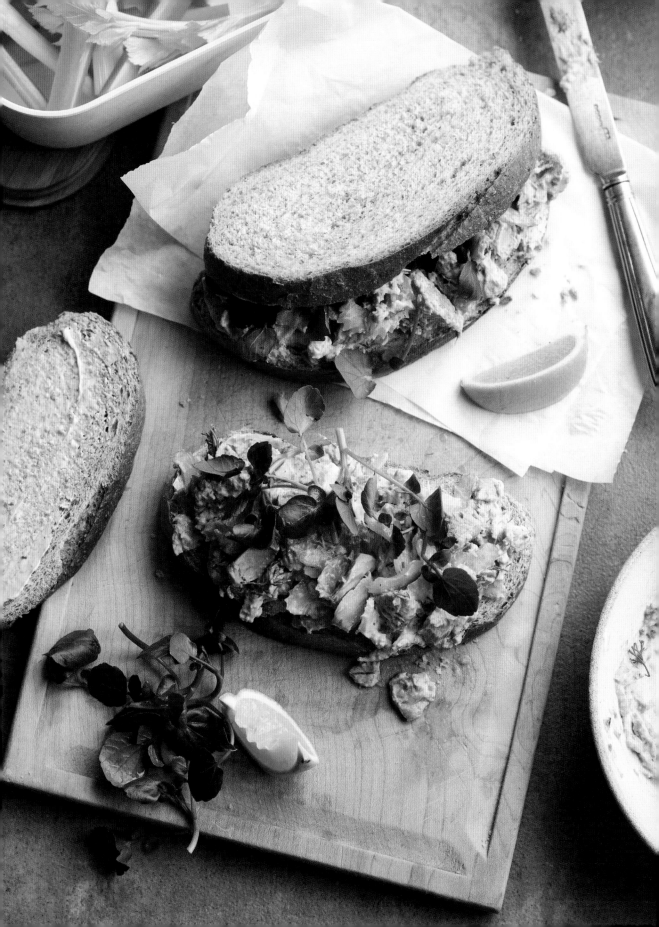

467
CALS

BBQ PORK KEBABS

PER SERVING | **467** CALS | **39G** PROTEIN | **16G** FAT | **42G** CARBS

prep 15 MINS · cook 12 MINS · FREEZE

SERVES 4

600g diced pork
2 tbsp Greek yogurt
juice of 1/2 lemon
4 sweet potato wraps
60g salad leaves

For the BBQ sauce:
50g brown sugar
100g tomato sauce
2 tsp cider vinegar
1/2 tbsp Worcestershire
    sauce
1 garlic clove, minced
1 tsp smoked paprika
1/2 tsp chilli powder
    (or more if you like
    it hot)
1/2 tsp salt
1/2 tsp mustard powder
1/4 tsp ground pepper

tip

*Soak the wooden skewers
in water for 1 hour before
using to avoid burning
when cooking.*

*These are great served with the super green salad
(see page 178) or naan breads (see page 184).*

1 To make the BBQ sauce, combine all the ingredients
in a saucepan. Bring to a boil over medium–high heat,
then reduce the temperature and cook the sauce until
it starts to reduce and thicken.

2 Divide the cubed pork into eight even portions and thread
onto short skewers. Brush with the BBQ sauce and allow
to marinate for at least 1 hour, or overnight is even better.

3 Heat up a cast iron griddle pan over high heat. Cook
the kebabs (in batches if needs be, depending on the size
of your pan) for about 12 minutes, turning every 2–3 minutes,
until the kebabs are golden and sticky and cooked through.
Brush with more BBQ sauce as you cook so they remain
glossy, but make sure all the sauce is exposed to the heat
as it's had raw meat in it.

4 While the meat is cooking, combine the yogurt and lemon
juice in a small bowl to make a sauce for drizzling.

5 Serve the pork kebabs with the sweet potato wraps, salad
leaves and lemony yogurt on the side so people can assemble
their own kebabs, or pack everything separately into meal
prep containers and assemble just before you eat.

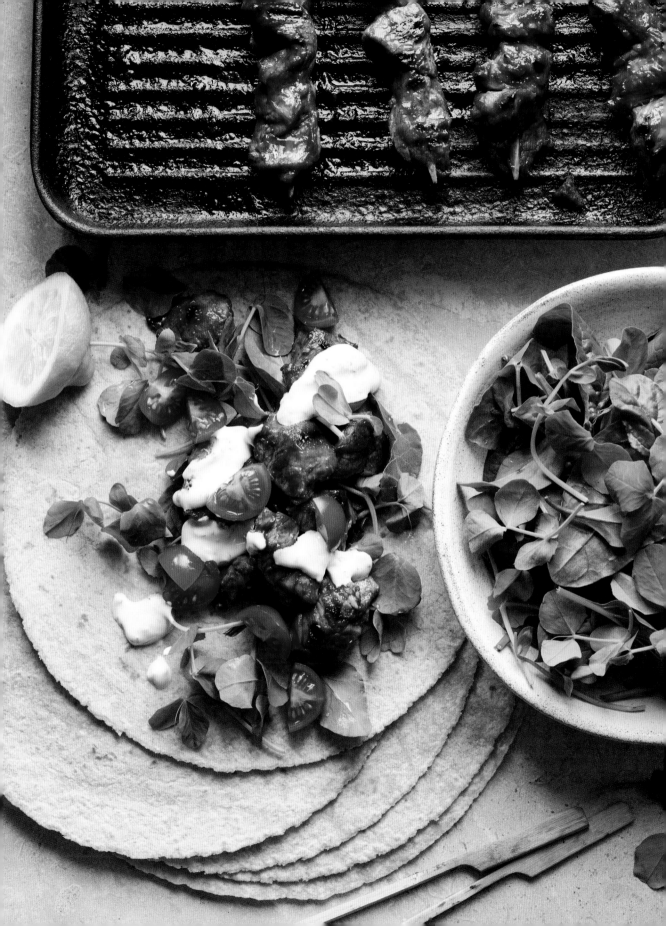

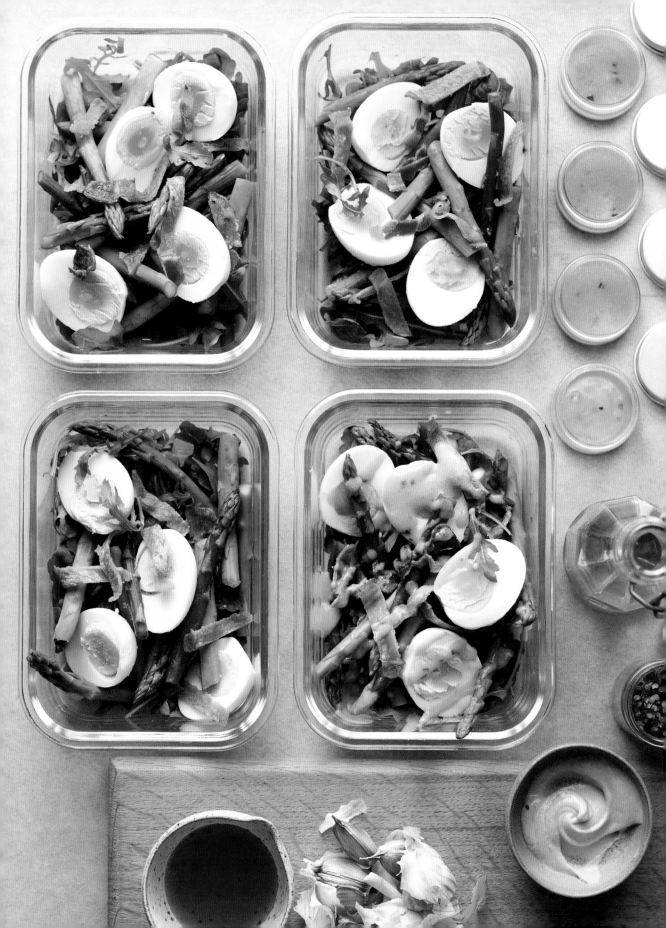

313
CALS

ROCKET, EGG AND ASPARAGUS SALAD

PER SERVING | **313** CALS | **24G** PROTEIN | **22G** FAT | **3G** CARBS

prep
15 MINS

cook
15 MINS

SERVES 4

8 eggs
3 tbsp olive oil, plus a
    drizzle for the bacon
4 slices back bacon
500g asparagus, ends
    trimmed and spears
    halved widthways
2 tbsp red wine vinegar
1 tbsp Dijon mustard
1 garlic clove, minced
a pinch of chilli flakes
50g rocket leaves
salt and pepper

tip

*Try visiting local farm
shops for fresher eggs.*

A meal prep that's great for a picnic on a nice afternoon walk.

1 Bring a pan of water to a rolling boil and add the eggs.
Boil for 6 minutes for soft yolks (slightly longer if you want the
yolks firmer), then drain immediately under cold running water.
Allow the eggs to cool a little before peeling and setting aside.

2 While the eggs are cooking, cook the bacon. Drizzle a tiny
bit of oil into a non-stick frying pan over high heat and fry
the bacon rashers until crisp. Once cool enough to handle,
chop them into small bits and set aside.

3 Bring a large pan of salted water to a boil. Drop in the
asparagus and boil for 3–4 minutes – make sure you don't
overcook it as you want a little crunch. Using a slotted spoon,
remove the asparagus from the boiling water and transfer
to a bowl of iced water to stop the cooking process.

4 In a small mixing bowl, combine the oil, vinegar, mustard,
garlic and chilli flakes. Season with salt and pepper and whisk
to combine.

5 Divide the rocket leaves between four plates or meal
prep containers and top with the asparagus spears. Sprinkle
over the bacon pieces and top with the hard-boiled eggs –
sliced in half if eating right away, but leave whole for meal
prep. Drizzle with vinaigrette or pop it into a little container
to add later. Great warm or cold.

496
CALS

CHEESY MEXICAN BEEF

PER SERVING | **496** CALS | **34G** PROTEIN | **9G** FAT | **68G** CARBS

prep
15 MINS

cook
30 MINS

FREEZE

SERVES 4

2 tsp olive oil
1 small red onion, sliced
2 garlic cloves, minced
1 red pepper, deseeded
  and diced
1 green pepper,
  deseeded and diced
400g very lean (4%)
  steak mince
260g easy-cook rice
1 x 400g tin chopped
  tomatoes
1¹/2–2 tbsp Mexican
  seasoning
1 beef stock cube
50g low-fat Cheddar
  cheese
salt and pepper
a handful of fresh
  coriander, to serve

*This brilliant, tasty one-pot dish will help you cut down
on your washing up as well as your calories.*

1 Heat the oil in a large pan over a medium heat, add the
onion, garlic and red and green peppers and fry for a minute.

2 Add the beef to the pan and cook for a few minutes until
nice and brown.

3 Add the rice, chopped tomatoes and Mexican seasoning
to the pan. Crumble the stock cube into a jug and add 500ml
boiling water from the kettle. Stir until the cube is dissolved,
then add the stock to the pan too. Lower the heat to low,
cover the pan with a lid and simmer for 20 minutes or so,
stirring frequently so it doesn't catch on the bottom of the
pan, until the rice is cooked and all the water is absorbed.

4 Taste and season with salt and pepper to taste. Top the
rice with cheese and pop the lid back on for a minute or so
for it to melt, then sprinkle with coriander leaves to serve.

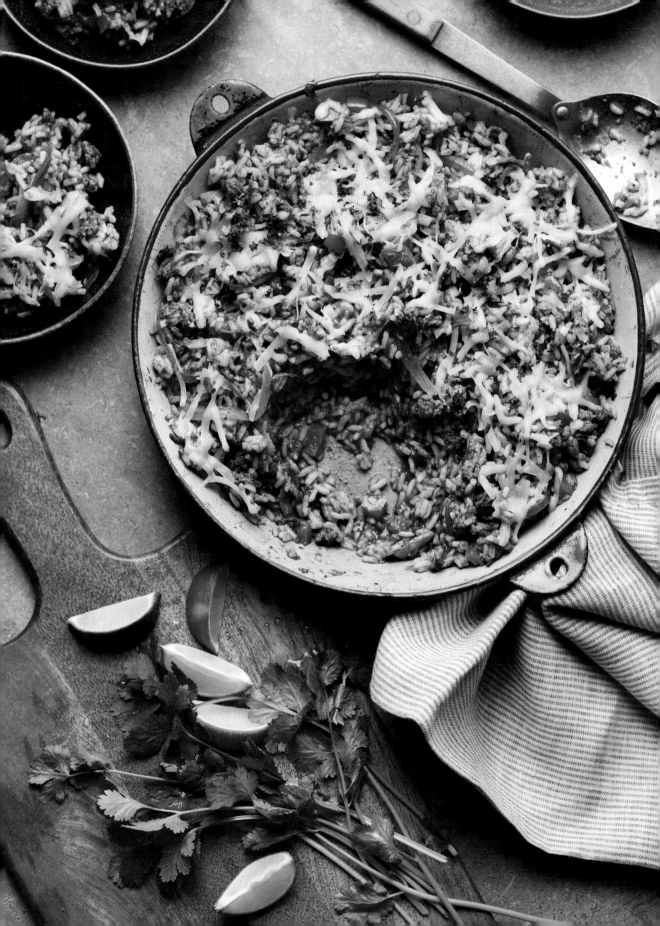

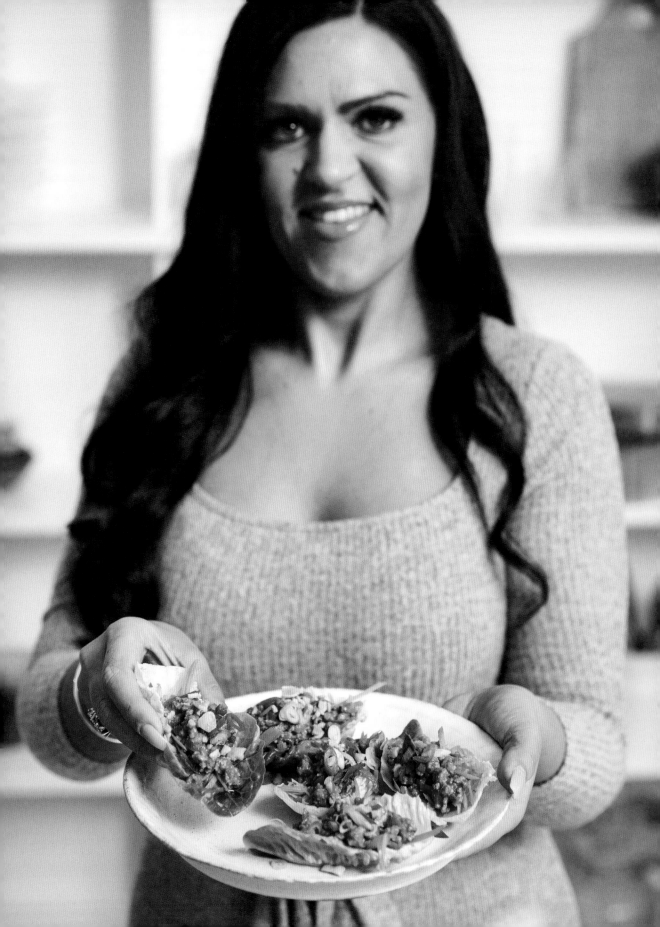

326
CALS

THAI TURKEY LETTUCE WRAPS

PER SERVING | **326** CALS | **39G** PROTEIN | **14G** FAT | **9G** CARBS

15 MINS   12 MINS   FREEZE

SERVES 4

60g smooth peanut butter
juice of 1 lime
3 tbsp dark soy sauce
1 tbsp rice vinegar
2 tsp sesame oil
½–1 red chilli, finely diced
   (optional)
1 tbsp olive oil
1 onion, finely sliced
3 garlic cloves, minced
1 tbsp Thai red curry paste
500g turkey breast mince
150g carrots, peeled and
   grated or shredded
1 large romaine lettuce
   or 2 little gem lettuces
a few crushed peanuts
   and sliced spring onions
   and chillies, to garnish

*The turkey filling freezes
really well without the
lettuce, so you can make
it in advance and freeze
in portions.*

*These are a great light lunch, or serve the turkey filling
in tortillas to make it more substantial.*

1 Add the peanut butter, lime juice, soy sauce, rice vinegar,
sesame oil and chilli, if using, to a large glass jar and shake
it up until smooth.

2 Put the olive oil in a large non-stick frying pan and fry
the onion for a good 5 minutes until softened. Add the
garlic and the curry paste and cook for 2–3 minutes longer.

3 Add the mince to the pan a little at a time to get some nice
brown colour on there. Scrape any crispy bits off the bottom
of the pan as it cooks. Once the mince is cooked, add the
carrot and the peanut sauce and stir in, cooking for another
1–2 minutes. Add a little splash of water if looking dry.

4 Break off the lettuce leaves from the head and fill them
with the turkey mixture. Sprinkle chopped peanuts and sliced
spring onions over the tops. I sometimes add a fresh sliced
chilli too – I like everything spicy.

447
CALS

PRAWN TACOS

PER SERVING | **447** CALS | **37G** PROTEIN | **13G** FAT | **41G** CARBS

prep 10 MINS   cook 5 MINS

SERVES 2

½ x 400g tin of black
  beans, drained
  and rinsed
4 spring onions,
  finely sliced
2 plum tomatoes, diced
1 red or green chilli,
  finely chopped, plus
  (optional) extra to serve
a small bunch of fresh
  coriander, chopped
1 tbsp olive oil
300g raw king prawns
½ tsp ground cumin
½ tsp smoked paprika
¼ tsp chilli powder
4 small tortillas
salt and pepper
2 tbsp soured cream,
  to serve

*Prawns are a great low-fat, flavour-packed alternative
to other meats usually found in tacos.*

1 Put the beans, spring onions, tomatoes, chilli and coriander
in a bowl with lots of seasoning and 1 tsp of the olive oil.
Toss together until well combined, then place to one side.

2 Drizzle the remaining olive oil over the prawns in a bowl,
sprinkle with the spices and toss to coat them all well. Cook
the prawns in two batches in a large non-stick frying pan over
high heat, until they are golden on the outside and cooked
through – about 3–4 minutes.

3 Meanwhile, heat up the tortillas on a griddle if possible,
to add some char lines, or use a microwave.

4 To assemble, top the tortillas with the bean mix, then
add the prawns and a blob of soured cream. I like to add
extra chilli to mine. If you are preparing this for meal prep,
keep the elements separate until ready to eat.

tip

*If you like, you can add a
little chorizo to this. Just
add it to the dry frying
pan and cook a little for
it to release its oils, then
add the prawns (no need
for the oil this time) and
cook them through.*

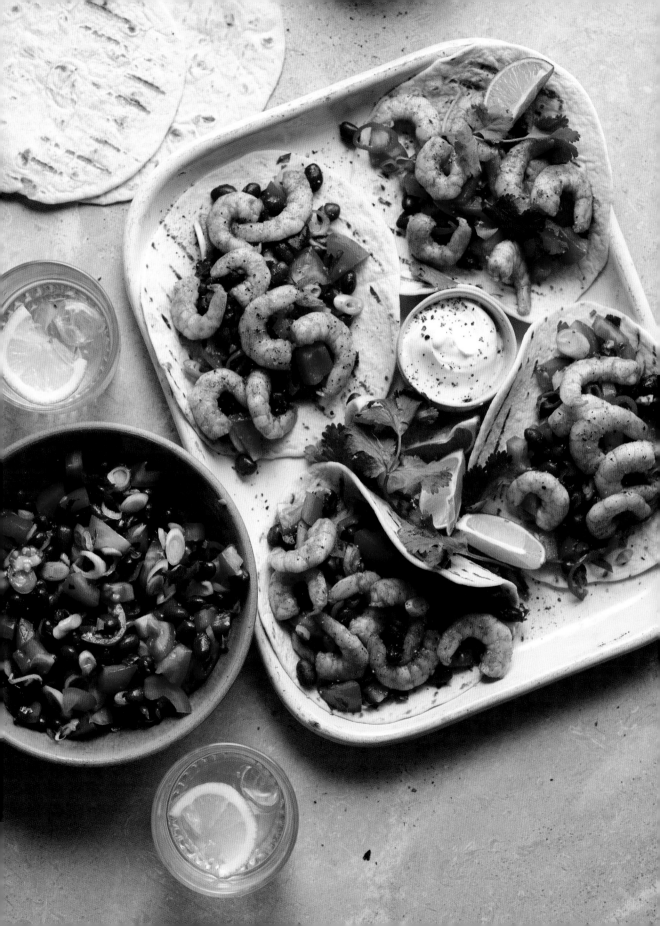

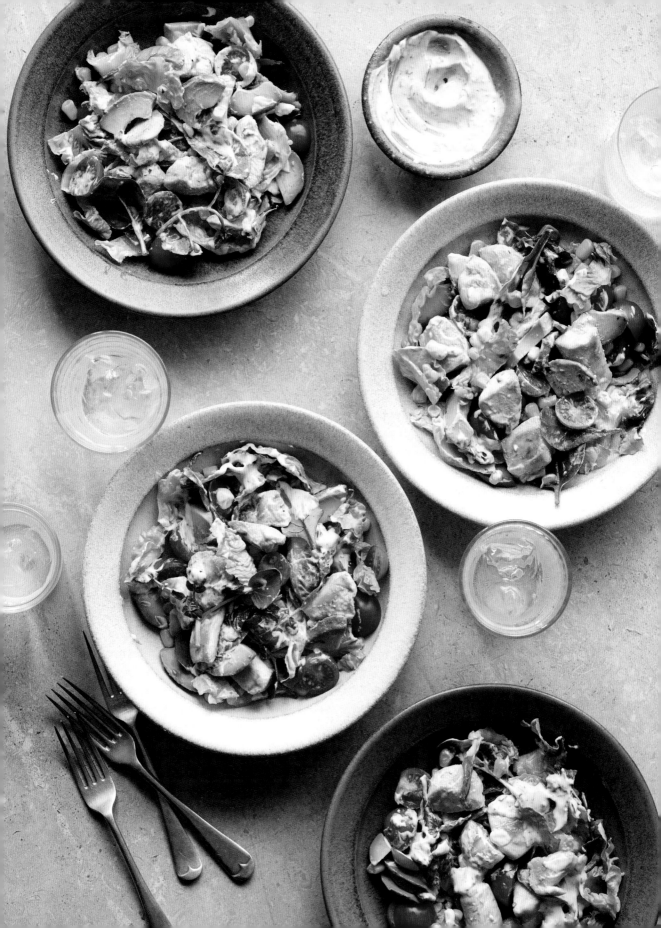

HEALTHY RANCH CHICKEN

PER SERVING | **330** CALS | **37G** PROTEIN | **14G** FAT | **11G** CARBS

15 MINS +
MARINATING   15 MINS

SERVES 4

500g chicken breasts,
    cut into bite-sized pieces
1 tbsp olive oil
a bag of mixed salad greens
    (or chopped lettuce)
½ small red onion,
    finely sliced
160g cherry tomatoes,
    halved
½ cucumber, sliced
120g drained tinned
    sweetcorn
1 avocado, peeled,
    pitted and sliced
    (see note in method)

For the ranch dressing:
250g fat-free Greek yogurt
2–3 garlic cloves, crushed
2 tsp lemon juice
1 tbsp Dijon mustard
1 tbsp chopped fresh
    parsley
1 tbsp chopped fresh dill
salt and pepper

*A super-quick light lunch, with a really punchy flavour from
the dressing, which leaves you feeling full and satisfied.*

1 Start with making the ranch dressing. Put all the ingredients
in a small jar, place the lid on, then shake to combine. If you
don't have an empty jam jar, use a small bowl and whisk
everything together.

2 Pour about one third of the dressing over the chicken and
allow it to marinate for at least 30 minutes. Place the chicken
and the remaining dressing in the fridge until ready to use.

3 Heat the oil in a large non-stick frying pan and add the
chicken. Cook until golden brown and cooked through,
about 6–7 minutes. You may need to do this in two batches,
depending on the size of your pan.

4 To assemble the salad, add the salad greens to a large
bowl. Top with remaining ingredients, then drizzle over
the dressing. If you are prepping this for later in the week,
don't slice the avocado yet – do it just before you eat it.
Store the dressing separately and just before serving,
toss with the dressing and enjoy!

397
CALS

BEEF KOFTA KEBABS WITH COUSCOUS

PER SERVING | **397** CALS | **40G** PROTEIN | **9G** FAT | **39G** CARBS

prep 20 MINS cook 10 MINS FREEZE

SERVES 4

For the koftas:
500g lean steak mince
40g dried breadcrumbs
½ red onion, grated
a handful of fresh parsley,
    finely chopped
3 garlic cloves,
    finely chopped
1 tsp black pepper
1 tsp chilli flakes
1 tsp ground coriander
½ tsp ground cumin
1 tsp smoked paprika
½ tsp salt
1 egg
a drizzle of olive oil,
    for cooking

For the couscous:
140g dried couscous
½ red onion, finely sliced
2 tbsp chopped fresh
    parsley
a few pomegranate seeds
salt and pepper

For the yogurt dressing:
200g low-fat Greek yogurt
1 garlic clove, crushed
1 tsp ground cumin
a squeeze of lemon
    juice, plus wedges
    for squeezing

Great for cooking on a BBQ in summer with friends and family. These also freeze really well – just defrost in the fridge the night before.

1 Combine all the kofta ingredients, except the oil, in a mixing bowl and mix everything together using your hands. It's time to get messy. When everything is mixed thoroughly, separate the mixture into eight equal portions. Roll each portion into a sausage shape and mould around a kebab stick.

2 Drizzle a griddle pan with a tiny bit of oil and heat over a medium–high heat. Cook the koftas on the griddle for about 10 minutes, turning every 2–3 minutes so they are evenly browned all over. You can also cook them under a grill or on the BBQ.

3 While the koftas are cooking, prepare the couscous. Put the dried couscous in a bowl and pour in 200ml boiling water from the kettle. Cover the bowl with a plate and leave for 5 minutes for the couscous to absorb the water. Once the 5 minutes are up, fluff up the couscous with a fork, stir in the onion and parsley and season with salt and pepper.

4 For the yogurt dressing, combine all the ingredients together in a small bowl and season with salt and pepper.

5 Divide the couscous between four meal prep containers and top each with two of the koftas and a sprinkle of pomegranate seeds. Drizzle the sauce over the top, or put in a separate little tub to take with you.

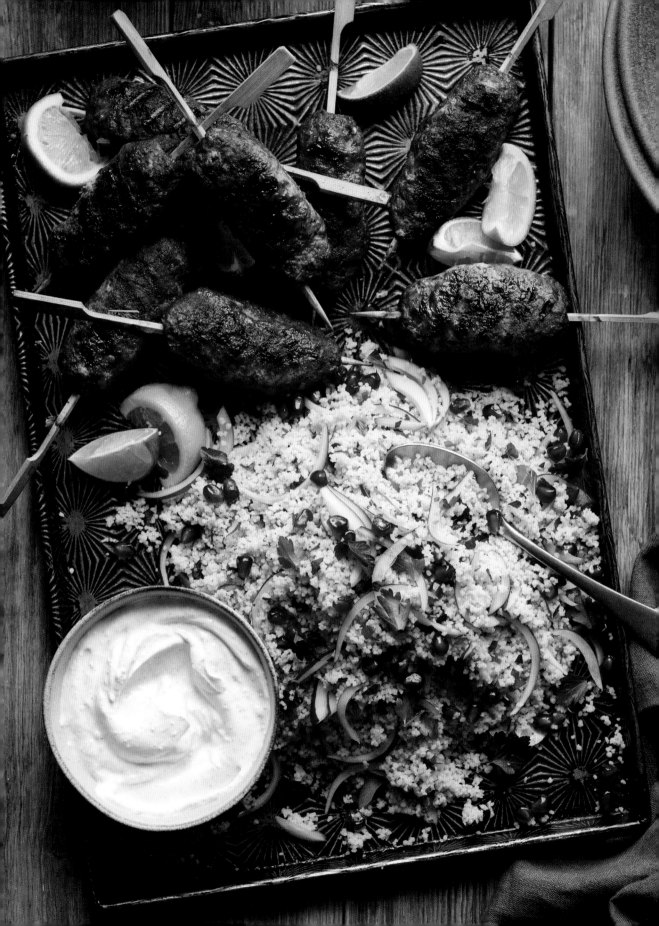

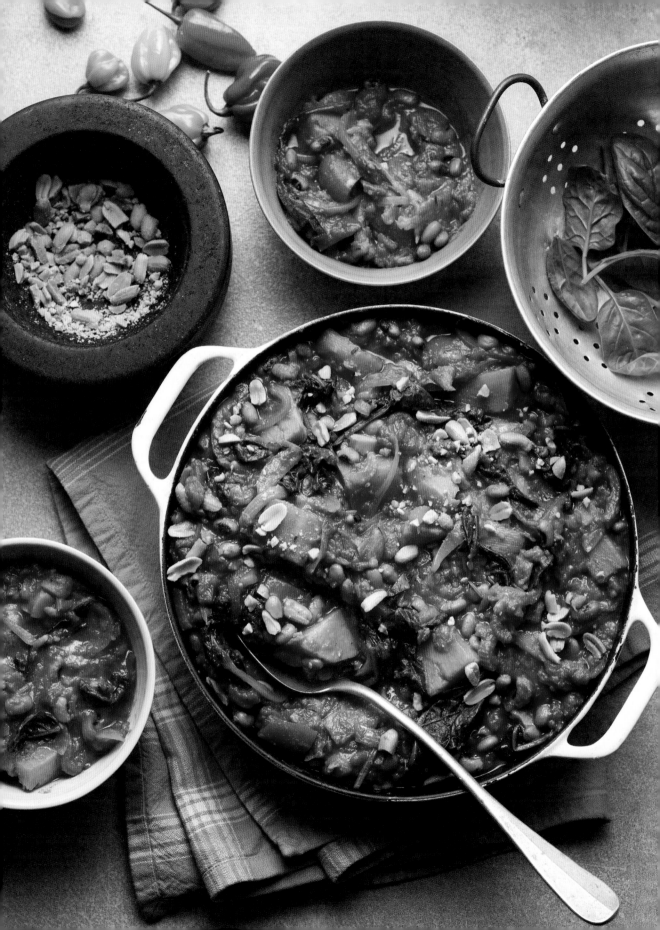

WEST AFRICAN VEGGIE STEW

PER SERVING | **449** CALS | **14G** PROTEIN | **13G** FAT | **63G** CARBS

10 MINS   3.5–7 HOURS   FREEZE

SERVES 6

1 tbsp olive oil
3 onions, sliced
1 tbsp dried thyme
4 garlic cloves, crushed
1–2 Scotch bonnet chillies (deseeded if you wish, depending how hot you want it), finely chopped
1.2kg sweet potatoes, peeled and chopped into 2.5cm chunks
3 x 400g tins chopped tomatoes
2 celery sticks, finely sliced
2 large red peppers, deseeded and chopped into large chunks
1 tsp ground ginger
1 tsp ground cumin
60g smooth peanut butter
2 x 400g tins black-eyed beans
150g young spinach leaves
salt and cayenne pepper
50g peanuts, crushed, to serve

Make this as hot as you dare! For a light tingle for wimps, use one deseeded Scotch bonnet; braver souls could go for two and leave the seeds in.

1 Heat the oil in a large non-stick frying pan and add the onions and thyme. Cook for a good 10 minutes until the onions are picking up some colour. Add the garlic and cook for a couple of minutes more, then transfer to the slow cooker.

2 Add the Scotch bonnet, sweet potatoes, tomatoes, celery, peppers and ground spices. Cook on HIGH for 3 hours, or on LOW for 6 hours.

3 Stir in the peanut butter and add the beans and cook for a final 30 minutes on HIGH or 1 hour on LOW. Five minutes from the end of cooking, stir in the spinach and allow it to wilt into the stew. Taste and season with salt and cayenne pepper and serve with crushed peanuts sprinkled over.

495 CALS

VEGGIE SINGAPORE NOODLES

PER SERVING | **495** CALS | **29G** PROTEIN | **18G** FAT | **51G** CARBS

prep
15 MINS

cook
10 MINS

SERVES 4

4 nests of rice
    vermicelli noodles
1 tbsp medium curry
    powder
2½ tbsp sesame oil
4 tbsp dark soy sauce
3 tbsp rice wine
1 tbsp vegetable oil
4cm piece of ginger,
    peeled and finely
    chopped
2 large garlic cloves,
    finely chopped
300g veggie protein pieces
120g shiitake mushrooms
1 medium-large carrot,
    peeled and finely sliced
1 red pepper, sliced
8 spring onions, sliced,
    white and green parts
    kept separate
1 small tin sliced water
    chestnuts, drained
100g baby corn, sliced
    diagonally
100g mangetout or sugar
    snap peas, halved if large
½ head Chinese leaf
    cabbage

These flavoursome noodles are packed with veg. You can use veggie protein pieces, as here, or chicken if you prefer, although the calorie count may differ.

1 Put the noodle nests in a bowl and pour over a kettle of boiling water so they are all submerged. Leave for 5 minutes until well softened, then drain and return to the now empty bowl. Stir in the curry powder, 1 tbsp sesame oil, 1 tbsp of the soy sauce and 1 tbsp hot water and stir well until the noodles are completely coated. Set aside.

2 In a jug, combine the remaining 3 tbsp soy sauce, the 3 tbsp rice wine and 2 tbsp water and set aside.

3 In a wok or large frying pan, heat the remaining sesame oil and the vegetable oil over high heat. Add your ginger and garlic and cook for a few seconds, then add the veggie protein. Cook for a couple of minutes until picking up some colour, then add the mushrooms, carrot, pepper, spring onion whites, water chestnuts and baby corn. Cook for a couple of minutes until softening, then add the mangetout and Chinese leaves. Cook for a minute, then pour over the liquid in the jug. Add the noodles and stir fry for a couple of minutes until everything is heated through.

4 Serve the noodles sprinkled with the spring onion greens, or pack into meal prep containers for another day.

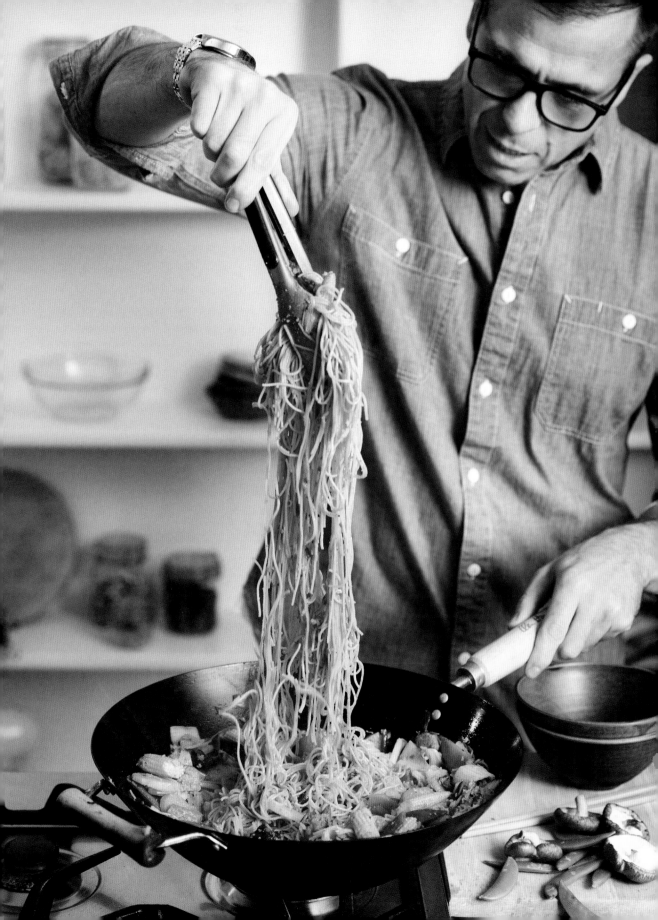

339 CALS

ROAST VEG AND PESTO POLENTA TART

PER SERVING | 339 CALS | 12G PROTEIN | 17G FAT | 33G CARBS

prep 20 MINS   cook 45 MINS   FREEZE

SERVES 4

low-calorie cooking
   oil spray
1 small aubergine, diced
1 courgette, diced
1 red pepper,
   cut into squares
1 yellow pepper,
   cut into squares
1 small red onion,
   cut into slim wedges
1 tbsp olive oil
1 veggie stock cube
150g quick polenta
50g Parmesan cheese,
   finely grated
½ recipe quantity Pesto
   (see page 68)
salt and pepper
fresh basil leaves,
   to serve (optional)

Cornmeal can make a great tart base, and is lower in calories than buttery pastry. Top it with delicious roasted veggies and a few blobs of pesto for a punch of flavour.

1 Preheat the oven to 200°C fan and spray a 23cm loose-based tart or pie tin with cooking spray.

2 Spread the veg out on a large baking tray and drizzle with the olive oil. Season with salt and pepper and toss everything to coat with oil. Roast for 30 minutes, or until everything is golden and tender.

3 Meanwhile, measure out 600ml water and get it boiling in a pan. Add the stock cube and stir until dissolved. Turn the heat down to medium so the water is at a gentle boil rather than rolling. With a wooden spoon in one hand and the polenta in the other, pour the polenta into the water in a thin and steady stream, beating all the time to avoid lumps. Add the grated Parmesan and keep cooking and stirring over the heat for about 5 minutes until the polenta is really thickening up. Pour the polenta into the tart tin and spread level, then pop it in the oven below the veggies. (Give the veggies a stir at this point as they are probably halfway through cooking by now.) Cook the tart base for 30 minutes, until firm and golden on top.

4 Once your tart base and veggies are all cooked, allow the base to cool for a couple of minutes, then remove it from the tin. Pile the veggies on top of the base and drizzle over the pesto. Garnish with extra basil leaves, if you like. If you are meal prepping this, keep the pesto in a separate sealed container and pour it over just before eating.

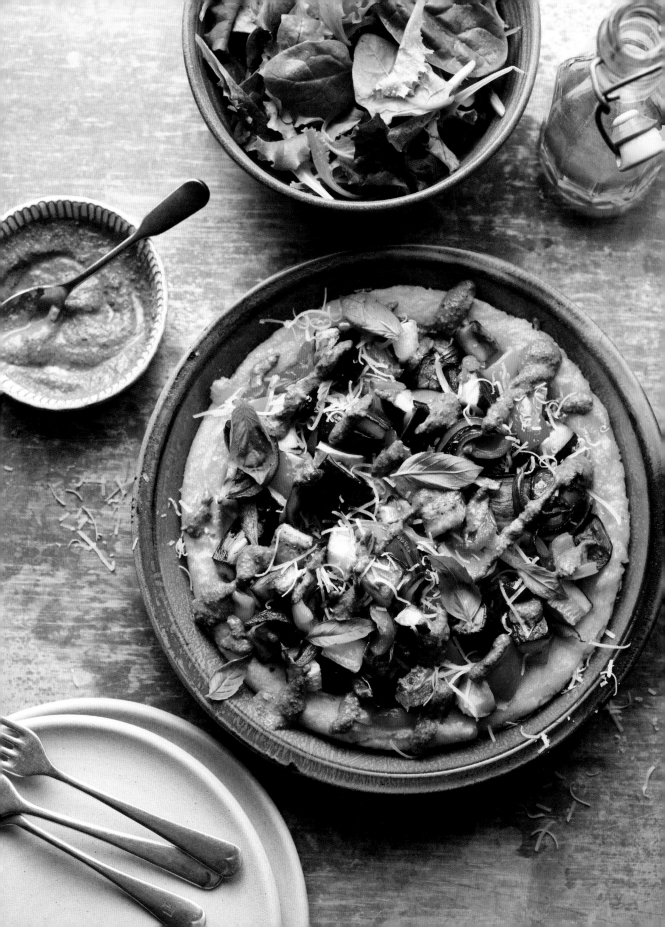

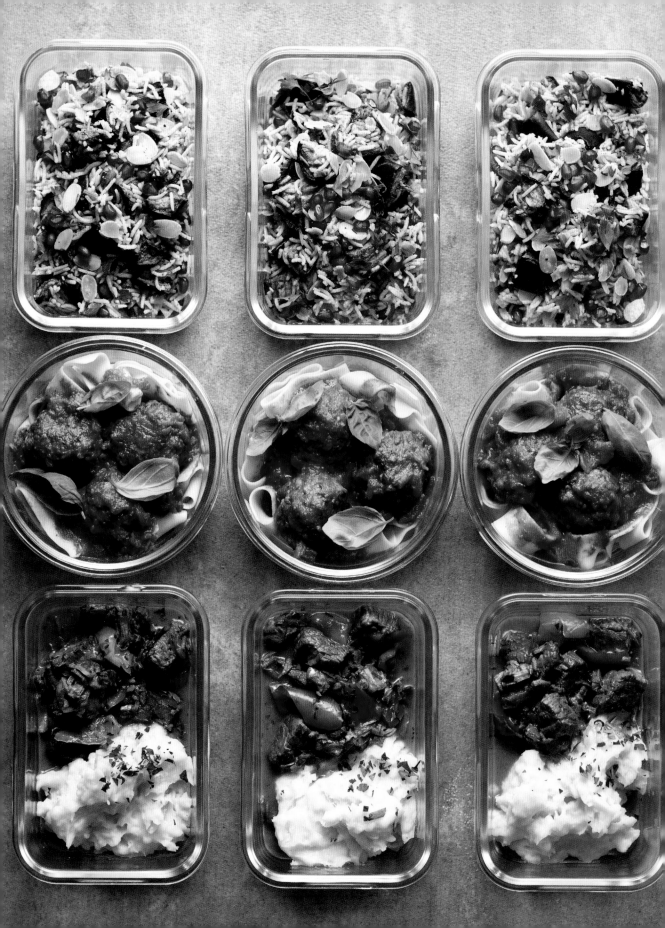

DINNER

475
CALS

ZINGER BURGER

PER SERVING | **475** CALS | **41G** PROTEIN | **18G** FAT | **38G** CARBS

prep
20 MINS

cook
20 MINS

FREEZE

MAKES 2

40g tortilla chips,
  crushed
1 egg
40g plain flour
1 tsp onion granules
1 tsp dried oregano
1 tsp chilli powder
1 tsp garlic granules
1 tsp paprika
2 chicken breasts
  (around 140g each)
low-calorie cooking
  oil spray

To assemble:
2 brioche buns,
  sliced in half
4 tsp 'lighter than light'
  mayonnaise
lettuce leaves
chilli sauce of your choice
  (I use zero calorie)

tip

*We find using the cheaper
brands of tortilla chips
gives a crunchier texture.*

*Brioche buns vary a lot in calories, so make sure you
check the packet. We use ones that are 157 calories
and a 'lighter than light' mayonnaise.*

1 Preheat the oven to 180°C fan.

2 Crush up the tortilla chips into little pieces and pop them
in a bowl, then put the egg and flour in two other separate
bowls (I use meal prep containers).

3 Season the crushed tortilla chips with the onion granules,
oregano, chilli powder, garlic granules and paprika and give
it a good mix.

4 Slice the chicken breast into strips about 2.5cm wide
(you should get three to four per breast). Coat each one
in flour, then dip it in the egg and then the crushed tortilla
mixture, making sure it is fully coated each time. Place on
a non-stick baking tray and repeat the process until the
chicken is all used up.

5 Spray each chicken strip with some low-calorie cooking
spray and bake for 18–20 minutes until the chicken is
cooked through.

6 While your chicken is cooking, toast your brioche buns
and spread 1 tsp of mayonnaise over the bottom half of
each one. Top with a few lettuce leaves. When the chicken
is done, divide the strips between each bun and top with
a chilli sauce of your choice. If you are meal prepping this,
toast the buns but don't add the mayo just yet. Keep
everything separate and assemble just before you eat.

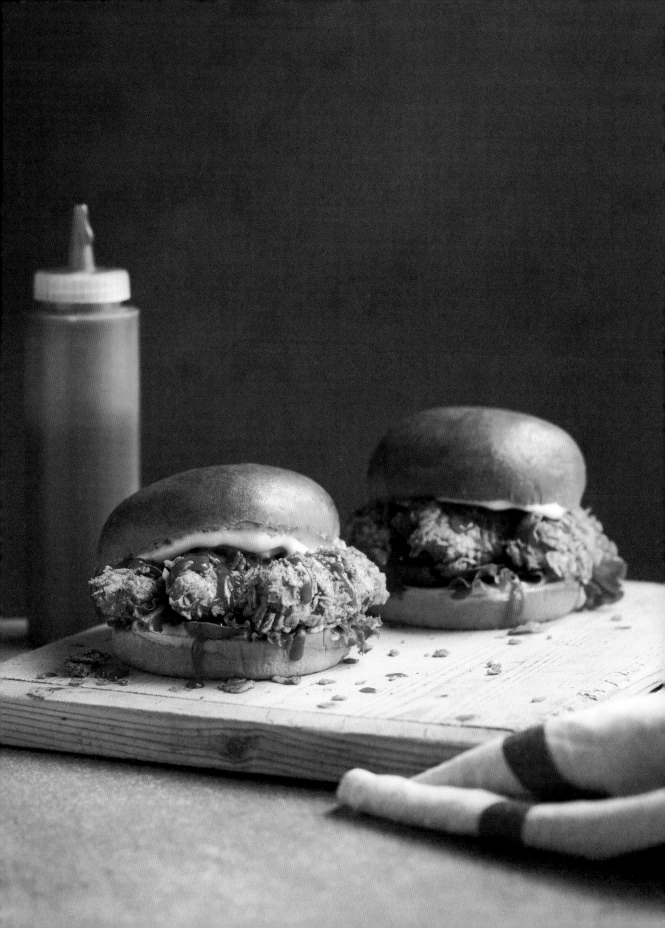

443 CALS

SHEPHERD'S PIE

PER SERVING | **443** CALS | **25G** PROTEIN | **20G** FAT | **39G** CARBS

25 MINS   50 MINS   FREEZE

SERVES 6

900g potatoes, peeled
   and chopped into chunks
2 tbsp olive oil
1 large onion,
   finely chopped
2 large carrots,
   finely chopped
1 garlic clove, minced
500g lean lamb mince
25g plain flour
1 tsp dried mixed herbs
1 tbsp tomato purée
1 x 400g tin chopped
   tomatoes
300ml lamb or beef stock
50g low-fat margarine
3 tbsp skimmed milk
1 tbsp butter, melted,
   for the top
salt and pepper
leafy greens, to serve
   (optional)

*Reheat these in the
oven in a glass meal
prep container for
the best results.*

*This meal prep brings back some childhood memories for
me, helping in the kitchen to mash the potatoes and lining
the top of the pie with a fork.*

1 Preheat the oven to 200°C fan.

2 Get a pan of salted water boiling and add the potatoes.
Cook for 15–20 minutes, or until soft.

3 Meanwhile, heat the oil in a non-stick frying pan and add
the onion and carrots. Cook for a good 5 minutes until really
beginning to soften. Add the garlic and cook for another
minute or so, then add the lamb mince and cook until
browned, stirring frequently.

4 Stir the flour and herbs into the mixture and cook for a
further 1 minute. Add the tomato purée, tomatoes and stock.
Stir, then allow to simmer and thicken for 10 minutes. Season
with salt and pepper, then spoon the mixture into an ovenproof
dish (or separate meal prep containers) and set aside.

5 By this time, the potatoes should be cooked. Drain them
and tip them back into the pan, adding the margarine and milk.
Season well, then mash until really smooth.

6 Spread the potatoes over the top of the lamb mixture and
crisscross the top with a fork to rough it up a little. Brush the
top of the pie with the melted butter. At this point, if being
used for meal prep, place in the fridge or freezer.

7 If you have just made the sauce and mash and it's all still
warm, cook the pie for about 20–25 minutes, just to get it hot
again and let the top go golden and crisp. If you are cooking
from chilled, it will probably need 45–50 minutes to get hot
again. You can also cook it now for meal prep and just rewarm
a portion in the microwave when you're ready to eat.

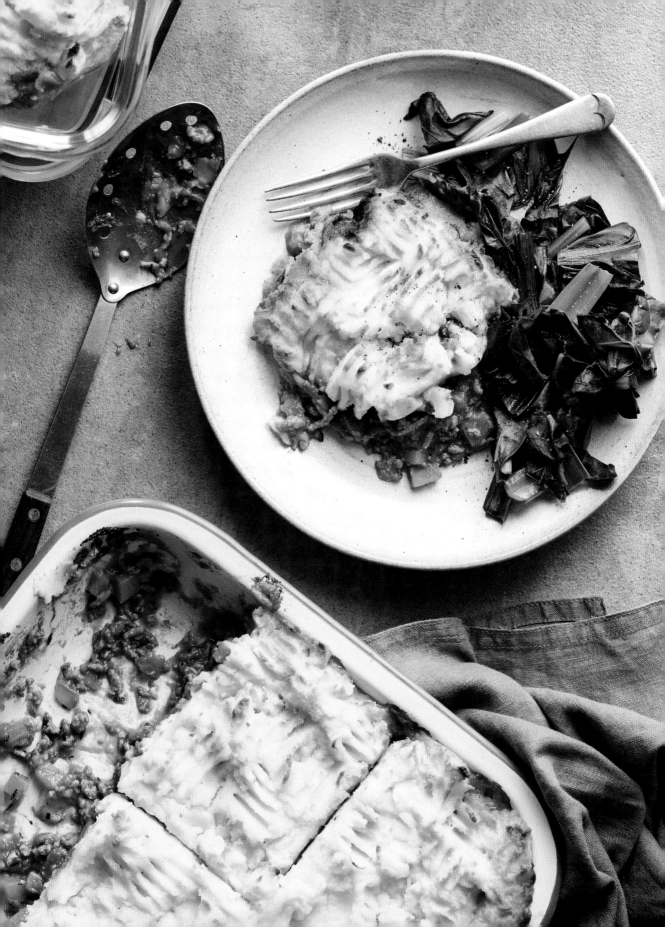

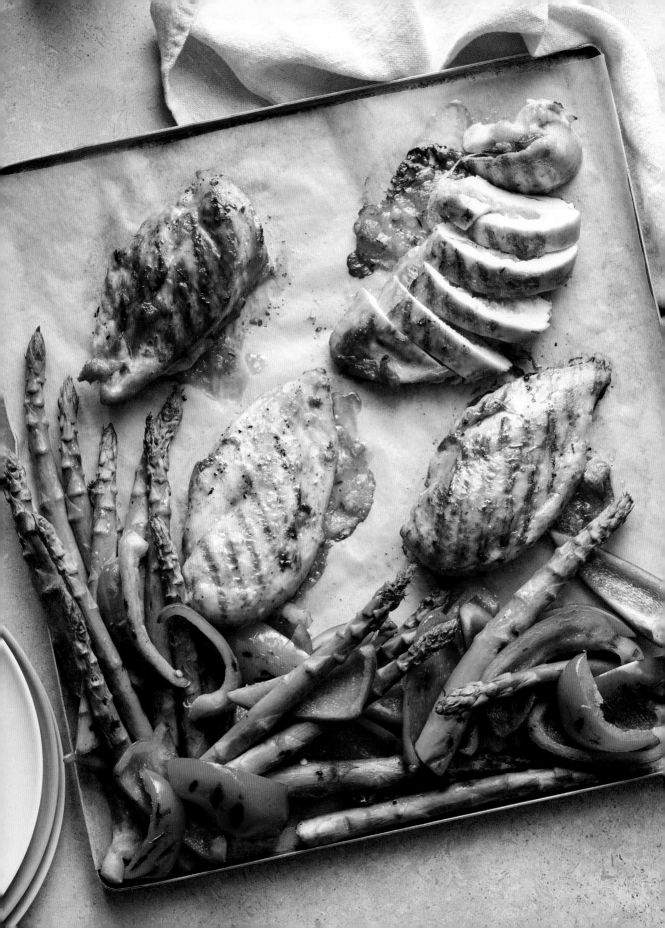

CHEESY STUFFED CHICKEN WITH GRIDDLED VEG

PER SERVING | 367 CALS | 53G PROTEIN | 13G FAT | 7G CARBS

prep 20 MINS   cook 25 MINS   FREEZE

SERVES 4

2 tbsp olive oil
1 small red onion, sliced
1 garlic clove, minced
1 tsp dried thyme
1/2 tsp dried rosemary
juice of 1 lemon or lime
4 chicken breasts
   (around 200g each)
100g reduced-fat
   mozzarella, grated
1 red pepper, deseeded
   and sliced
1 green pepper,
   deseeded and sliced
400g asparagus
salt and pepper

tip

A griddle pan is a great investment to add extra flavour and colour without adding extra calories.

This high-protein, low-carb meal is one of my favourites for after exercise. Charring the chicken and veg in the griddle pan adds tons of flavour.

1 Preheat the oven to 200°C fan and line a baking tray with foil or non-stick baking paper.

2 Heat 1 tbsp of the oil in a non-stick frying pan. Add the onion and cook for a few minutes until softened. Add the garlic and dried herbs and squeeze in the lemon juice. Cook for a few more minutes until the onion is well softened, then season to taste with salt and pepper.

3 Slice each chicken breast horizontally along its side to create a pouch, cutting in more deeply in the middle in order to create a deep pocket. Stir the grated cheese into the onion mixture and stuff each breast with a quarter of the mixture.

4 Heat up a cast iron griddle pan, if you have one, over high heat, or just use a heavy frying pan. Drizzle the griddle with a little oil and place the chicken breasts on the griddle. Cook for a few minutes on each side, or until charred lines have appeared. Using tongs, transfer the chicken breasts to the prepared baking tray and place in the preheated oven. Cook for about 15 minutes, or until the breast is fully cooked through and the cheese has melted.

5 Meanwhile, toss the sliced peppers and asparagus with the remaining oil in a bowl and season well with salt and pepper. Cook the vegetables, in batches if needs be, on the hot griddle, until charred and softened.

6 Serve the cheesy chicken with the veg, or divide between meal prep containers to enjoy later in the week.

498
CALS

TURKEY MEATBALL PASTA

PER SERVING | **498** CALS | **47G** PROTEIN | **10G** FAT | **53G** CARBS

20 MINS   30 MINS   FREEZE

SERVES 4

450g lean turkey mince
1 tsp chilli flakes
1 onion, finely chopped
2 garlic cloves, minced
2 tbsp fresh parsley,
   finely chopped
1 medium egg,
   lightly beaten
1 tbsp skimmed milk
60g breadcrumbs
40g Parmesan cheese,
   finely grated
1 tbsp olive oil
100ml chicken stock
400g passata
1 x 400g tin chopped
   tomatoes
200g dried
   pappardelle pasta
salt and pepper
fresh basil leaves,
   to garnish

My take on a classic Italian dish. Using lean turkey instead of beef keeps calories down but doesn't compromise on flavour.

1 In a large mixing bowl, combine the turkey mince, chilli flakes, onion, garlic, parsley, egg, milk, breadcrumbs, and Parmesan cheese. Mix it well until all the ingredients are well combined. Divide the mixture into 12 even portions and roll in balls using slightly wet hands.

2 Add the olive oil to a non-stick frying pan on medium–high heat and brown the meatballs in two batches, so they are in a single layer and don't touch each other. Fry them for about 1–2 minutes, turning over often, until they get a nice brown colour all over, then remove from the pan.

3 Add the chicken stock to the pan and scrape any browned bits from the bottom of the pan. Add the passata and chopped tomatoes and mix. Bring it to the boil and let it simmer for about 5–10 minutes, until thickened. Season to taste with salt and pepper.

4 Transfer the meatballs back to the pan, cover with a lid and cook for about 10 minutes. Meanwhile, cook the pappardelle according to the packet instructions, then drain.

5 Divide the pasta between pasta bowls or meal prep containers and top with the meatballs and sauce. Garnish with basil leaves, to serve.

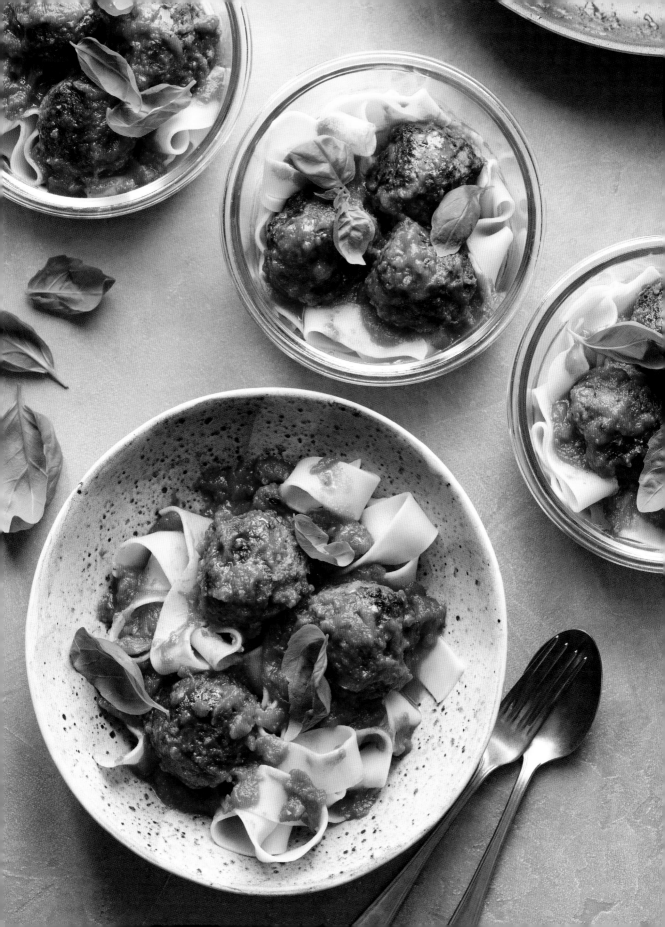

482
CALS

BAKED BUTTERNUT AND SAGE RISOTTO

PER SERVING | **482** CALS | **12G** PROTEIN | **8G** FAT | **86G** CARBS

prep
20 MINS

cook
1 HOUR

FREEZE

SERVES 6

1 medium-large butternut squash, peeled, deseeded, and cut into 2cm cubes (about 800g prepared weight)
2 red onions, sliced into thin wedges
2 tbsp olive oil
4 shallots, finely chopped
4 garlic cloves, minced
500g Arborio risotto rice
1.4 litres vegetable stock
1 tbsp chopped fresh sage
50g Parmesan, finely grated
20g fresh parsley, chopped
salt and pepper
a drizzle of balsamic glaze, to serve

tip

If you like, fry off some diced chorizo in a dry pan and sprinkle it over the top. Don't forget to weigh it and add the calories.

It was a neighbour of mine that suggested this recipe to me and once I made it, it soon became a household favourite. Very filling too.

1 Preheat the oven to 200°C fan.

2 Tip the butternut squash and onions onto two baking trays and drizzle each tray with ½ tbsp oil. Season and toss to coat everything in the oil. Roast for 25 minutes, or until the squash is tender. Once the veg is out of the oven, turn the oven down to 160°C fan.

3 Add the remaining oil to a large ovenproof casserole dish or Dutch oven and cook the shallots and garlic over a low heat for 3–4 minutes until softened. Add the rice and cook for 1–2 minutes, then add the stock and sage and stir everything together. Pop a lid on the pan and transfer it to the oven. Bake for 30 minutes, until the rice is tender and the risotto is thickened but still quite oozy.

4 Stir the grated Parmesan, roasted vegetables and parsley into the risotto and season with salt and pepper.

5 Divide the risotto between meal prep containers and allow to cool. Reheat in the microwave and drizzle the risotto with balsamic glaze to serve. Top with additional chopped fresh parsley, if you like.

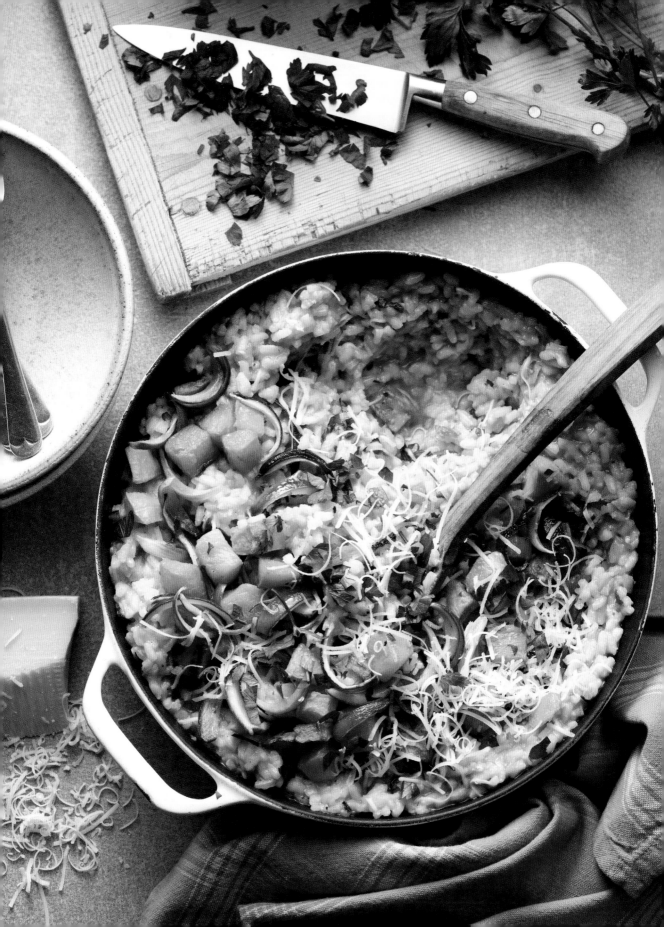

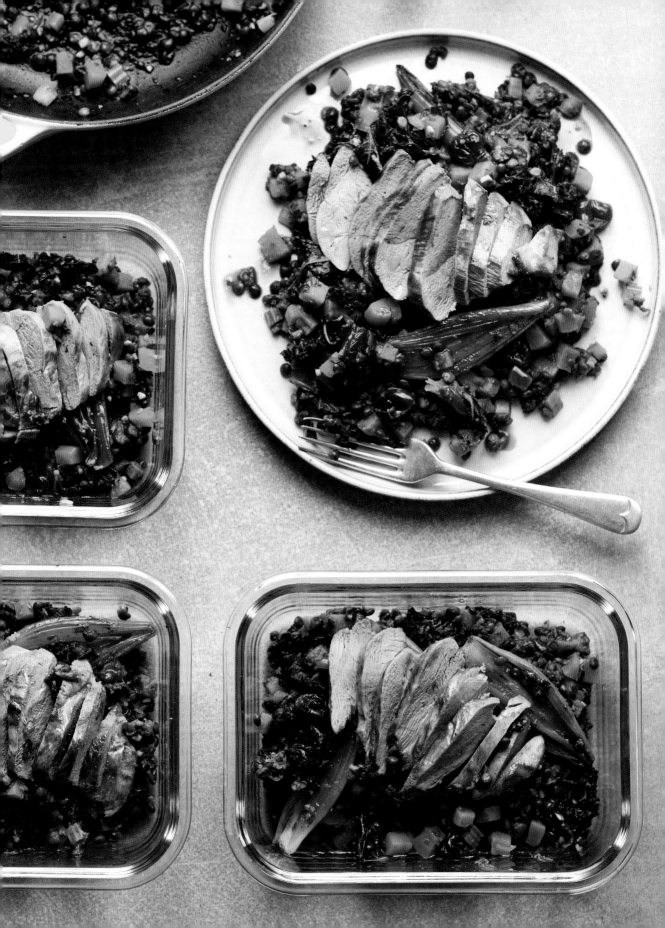

493 CALS

DUCK WITH LENTILS AND CHERRIES

PER SERVING | **493** CALS | **43G** PROTEIN | **15G** FAT | **42G** CARBS

prep **20 MINS** | cook **1 HOUR** | **FREEZE**

SERVES 4

1 tbsp olive oil
4 duck breasts,
    skin removed
300g banana (long)
    shallots, peeled and
    halved (or quartered
    if really large)
3 garlic cloves,
    finely chopped
1 tbsp finely chopped
    fresh rosemary
2 carrots, peeled and diced
2 celery sticks, diced
1 chicken stock pot
180g dried Puy lentils
1/4 tsp ground cinnamon
1 tsp Worcestershire sauce
60g dried cherries
100g chopped kale
salt and pepper

Duck can be a lean and healthy meat if you remove the thick layer of fatty skin, and the meat is still delicious. You can ask your butcher to do this, if you'd prefer.

1 Heat the oil in a large casserole over a high heat and brown the duck breasts on all sides until they are picking up a bit of colour. Remove from the pan and set aside, leaving the oil in the pan. Turn the heat down to medium–low and cook the shallots for a good 6-7 minutes, until picking up some colour and softening. Add the garlic, rosemary, carrots and celery to the pan and cook for 5 more minutes.

2 Dissolve the stock pot in 600ml boiling water, then add to the pan along with the lentils, cinnamon and Worcestershire sauce. Mix well, then pop the lid on the pan and simmer for 30 minutes, stirring occasionally.

3 Once the 30 minutes are up, stir the dried cherries and chopped kale into the mixture and season well with salt and pepper. If the mixture is looking dry, add a splash more hot water from the kettle. Return the duck breasts to the pan, laying them on top, and put the lid back on. Cook for a final 10 minutes until the duck is cooked throughout, but still a bit pink in the middle, and the lentils and vegetables are tender.

4 Slice the duck breasts and eat immediately, or divide between meal prep containers to be quickly reheated in the microwave when needs be.

391 CALS

SWEET POTATO CURRY

PER SERVING | **391** CALS | **11G** PROTEIN | **13G** FAT | **53G** CARBS

prep 10 MINS — cook 25 MINS — FREEZE

SERVES 4

2 tbsp coconut oil
1 onion, finely sliced
2 garlic cloves, crushed
2 tbsp tomato purée
2 tsp cumin seeds
1½ tsp mustard seeds
1 tbsp medium curry powder
600ml vegetable stock
1 x 400g tin chopped tomatoes
4 medium sweet potatoes, peeled and cut into 3cm chunks
100g red lentils
1 x 200ml tin light coconut milk
salt and pepper
a small handful of fresh coriander leaves, to garnish
natural yogurt and naan bread, to serve, or rice if you prefer (optional)

Social media followers have been begging us for this recipe for quite a while. A delicious curry that will appeal to both meat eaters and vegetarians.

1 Heat up the coconut oil in a large pan over low-medium heat, add the onion and sauté for a good 5 minutes until the onion is softened. Add the garlic, tomato purée, cumin and mustard seeds and the curry powder and cook for another minute or so.

2 Next, add your vegetable stock and chopped tomatoes and bring to the boil, then add the sweet potato and lentils and reduce to simmer. Cook for about 15 minutes, until the lentils have cooked and thickened the curry and the sweet potato is tender. Add the coconut milk at the last minute and cook just to heat through. Taste and season with salt and pepper.

3 Divide the curry between four plates or meal prep containers and garnish with fresh coriander. Eat on its own or it's great served with Greek yogurt, fresh naan bread or just rice, depending on how many calories you have to play with.

tip

Don't overcook the sweet potatoes, as they will turn to mush when reheated.

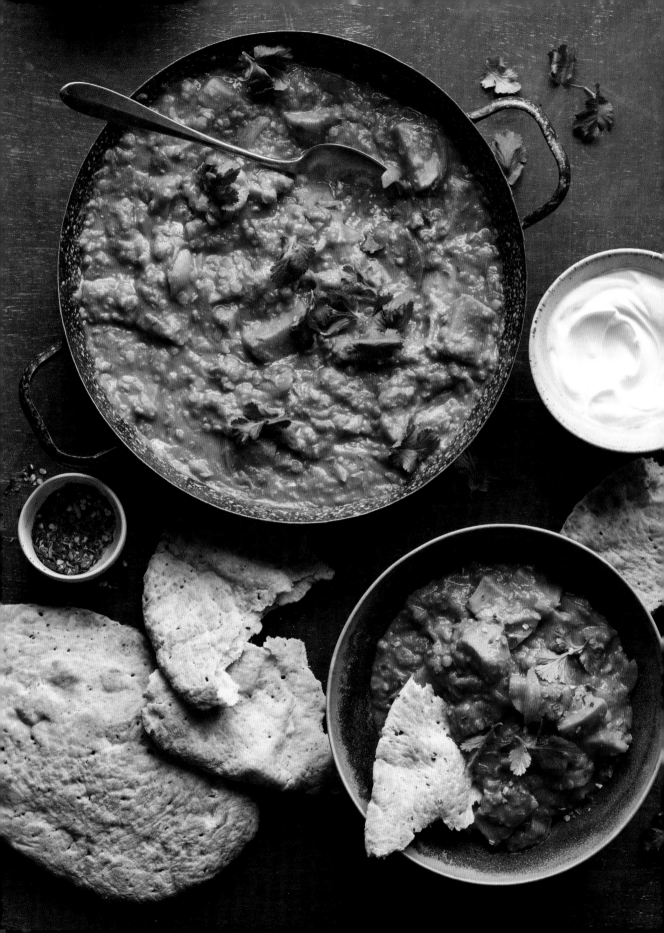

490 CALS

AUBERGINE PILAF

PER SERVING | **490** CALS | **10G** PROTEIN | **21G** FAT | **61G** CARBS

prep 20 MINS   cook 30 MINS   FREEZE

SERVES 4

For the aubergines:
2 aubergines, diced
　into 1.5cm chunks
2 tbsp olive oil
1 tsp ground coriander
1 tsp ground cumin
½ tsp ground cinnamon

For the rice:
30g flaked almonds
2 tbsp olive oil
1 large onion, finely diced
2 large garlic cloves,
　finely chopped
1½ tsp ground coriander
1½ tsp ground cumin
20g butter
250g basmati rice
700ml hot veg stock
a small handful of fresh
　parsley, roughly chopped
40g pomegranate seeds
salt and pepper

This colourful Middle Eastern dish is packed with flavour from the spices. Some people worry about reheating rice, but it's fine as long as you make sure it is chilled quickly after cooking and kept in the fridge.

1 Preheat the oven to 200°C fan.

2 Tip the aubergine cubes onto a baking tray and drizzle with the olive oil. Sprinkle over the spices and toss to coat well. Roast for 20–25 minutes, stirring halfway through, until soft and golden.

3 At the same time as the aubergine is cooking, toast the almonds. Tip them onto a baking tray and toast in the oven for 5 minutes, then remove and set aside.

4 While the aubergine is cooking, add the 2 tbsp olive oil to a large heavy-based saucepan or casserole and add the onion. Cook for a good 10 minutes over a low-medium heat until really well softened. Add the garlic and spices and cook for another couple of minutes. Add the butter and let it melt in the pan, then stir in the rice and leave to cook for 30 seconds or so. Pour in 600ml of the stock and stir well, then pop the lid on that pan and cook for 15 minutes. Check and if the rice is sticking to the pan, add a little more of the stock. Turn the heat off and leave it for another 10 minutes with the lid on – don't remove the lid at this point as the rice will keep cooking and go fluffier with the steam.

5 Stir the roasted aubergine and the parsley into the pilaf then season well with salt and pepper. Divide it between plates or meal prep containers and top with the pomegranate seeds and toasted flaked almonds.

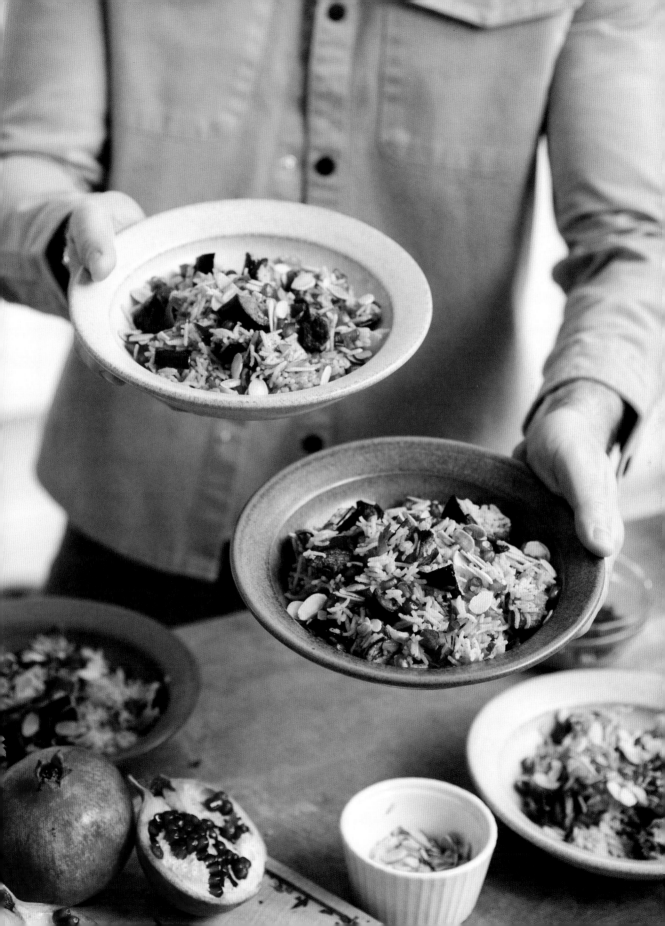

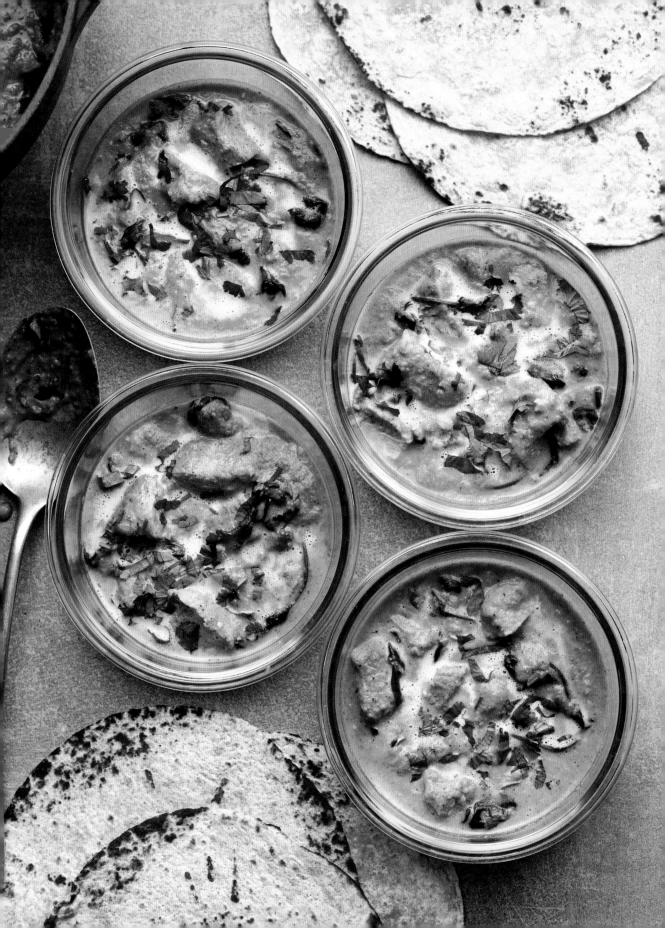

340
CALS

SLOW COOKER TURKEY KORMA

PER SERVING | **340** CALS | **39G** PROTEIN | **16G** FAT | **8G** CARBS

10 MINS   4 HOURS   FREEZE

SERVES 6

1 tbsp olive oil
400g diced onions (about
    3 medium–large onions)
1 tsp sugar
2 garlic cloves,
    roughly chopped
1 tbsp ground coriander
1 tbsp ground cumin
1 tsp ground turmeric
1 tsp mild chilli powder
1 tsp paprika
1 x 400g tin full-fat
    coconut milk
900g turkey breast
    steaks, diced
a squeeze of lemon juice
1 tbsp ground almonds
2 tsp garam masala
200g fresh spinach leaves
salt and pepper
chopped fresh coriander
    leaves, to garnish

A delicious milder curry, for the flavour lovers that like to enjoy a curry without the extra spice and heat.

1 Add the oil to a frying pan on a medium heat. Add in the onions and sugar and cook for about 5 minutes until really softening, then add the garlic and cook for a further 1 minute.

2 Add the coriander, cumin, turmeric, chilli powder and paprika to the pan, season with salt and pepper and stir in. Cook the mixture for about 2–3 minutes more, then transfer it to a blender. Reserve 3 tbsp of the coconut milk, then add the rest into the blender and blend until smooth.

3 Add the turkey breast and the spice mixture to a slow cooker and cook on LOW for 4 hours. Halfway through cooking, stir in the lemon juice, ground almonds and garam masala.

4 Once cooked, stir in the spinach and allow to wilt in the hot curry for a few minutes.

5 Divide the curry between meal prep containers and drizzle with the remaining coconut milk and sprinkle with fresh coriander. Serve with some rice or naan breads.

492
CALS

PIZZA PASTA BOWLS

PER SERVING | **492** CALS | **18G** PROTEIN | **25G** FAT | **46G** CARBS

prep
15 MINS

cook
12 MINS

FREEZE

SERVES 6

350g spinach trottole pasta
100g cherry tomatoes,
    sliced in half
50g jalapeño peppers
    (optional)
24 mini mozzarella pearls
100g mini pepperoni circles
1 red pepper, diced
1 green pepper, diced
40g low-fat Parmesan
    cheese, grated (we use
    a super low-fat one)
1 handful of fresh basil,
    chopped

For the dressing:

90ml extra virgin
    olive oil
60ml red or white
    wine vinegar
1 tsp sugar
1 tsp dried oregano
½ tsp garlic granules
a pinch of chilli flakes
salt and pepper

*Want to enjoy the taste of pizza without the bread?
Then this meal prep is ideal for you.*

1 Bring a pan of salted water to the boil and cook the
pasta according to the packet instructions until al dente.
Drain and run the pasta under cold water to cool down
completely and stop it cooking. Once drained, add to
a large mixing bowl.

2 In a glass jar, combine all the ingredients for the dressing
and season well with salt and pepper. Shake well.

3 Add the tomatoes, jalapeños, if using, mozzarella pearls,
pepperoni, peppers, Parmesan cheese and basil to the
pasta and mix. Pour the dressing over and mix well.

4 Divide the pasta between plates or meal prep containers.
Enjoy cold or warmed up in the microwave.

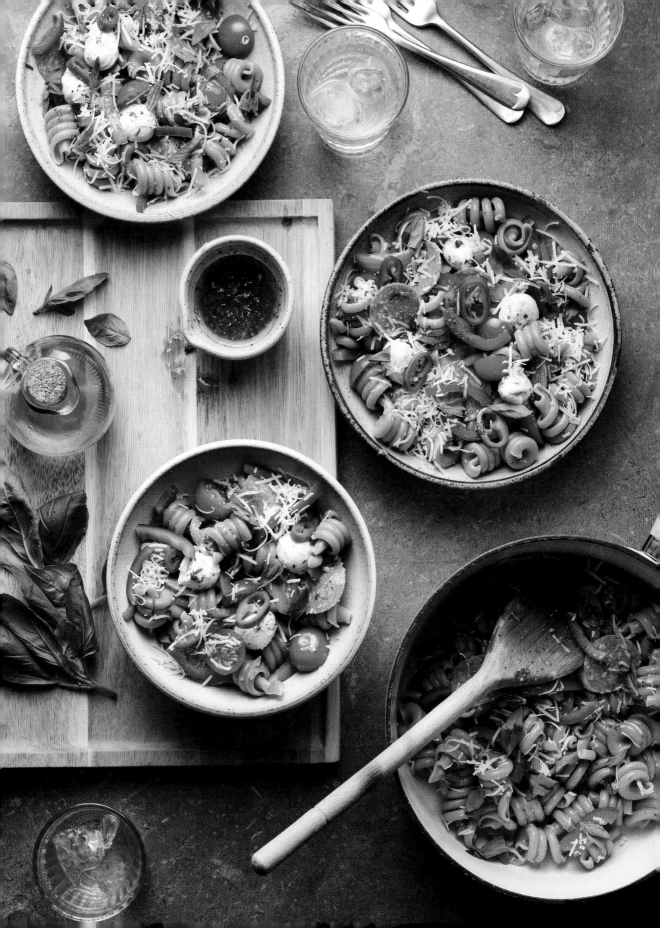

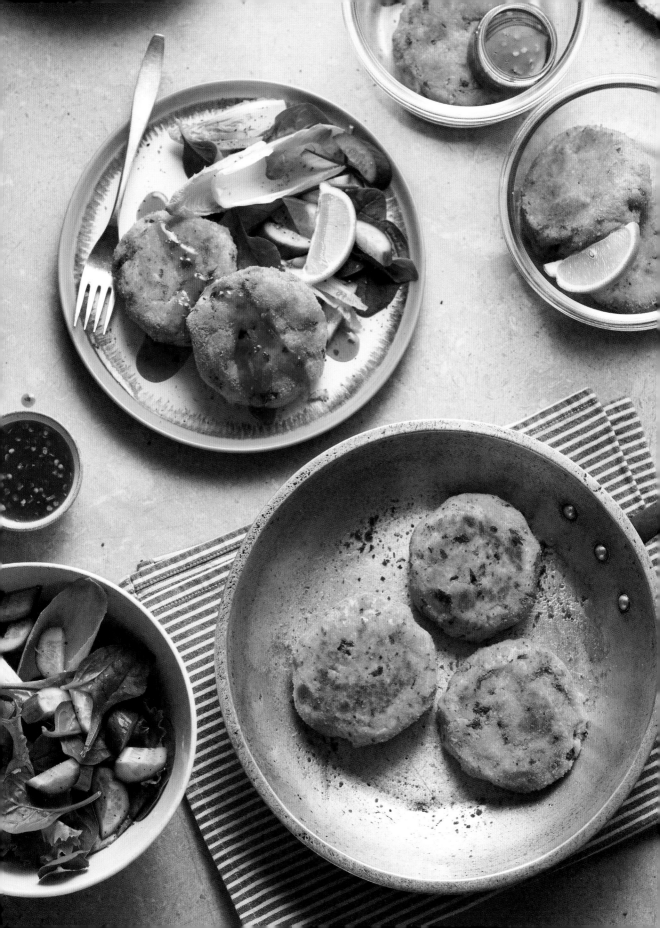

SALMON FISHCAKES WITH SWEET CHILLI SAUCE AND SALAD

PER SERVING | **460** CALS | **28G** PROTEIN | **11G** FAT | **60G** CARBS

20 MINS +
CHILLING **40 MINS** **FREEZE**

SERVES 4

800g potatoes
320g salmon
a handful of fresh flatleaf
   parsley, finely chopped
1 tsp garlic powder
40g plain flour
2 eggs, beaten
80g dried golden
   breadcrumbs
low-calorie cooking
   oil spray
salt and pepper

To serve:
1 lemon, sliced into wedges
a bag of mixed salad leaf
sweet chilli sauce (I use
   zero calorie)

*Make sure to buy the
golden breadcrumbs,
as these are what give
the fishcakes the lovely
golden colour.*

Salmon fishcakes are another meal prep that can be enjoyed hot or cold.

1 Peel and chop the potatoes into chunks. Place in a pan of salted water and boil for 20–25 minutes until soft. Once cooked, drain well, season with salt and pepper and mash until there are no lumps. Put the potato in a large mixing bowl.

2 Meanwhile, put the salmon in a microwaveable bowl and cover. Microwave for 3–4 minutes until just cooked. Alternatively, you can poach the salmon or bake it in the oven until just cooked. Once cooked, flake the fish into large pieces and add to the bowl with the potatoes. Add the parsley and garlic powder and mix really thoroughly. Taste and adjust the seasoning, adding more if you think it needs it. Allow the mixture to cool, then cover the bowl and place it in the fridge, giving it at least 2 hours to chill.

3 To assemble your fishcakes, divide the chilled mixture into eight equal portions. Tip the flour onto a work surface, turn the portions onto it and shape them into eight patties.

4 Put the beaten eggs in a shallow bowl and the breadcrumbs in another bowl. One by one, turn the patties over in the egg, then in the breadcrumbs to coat them all over.

5 Spray a hot pan with cooking spray, and fry over medium heat for 2–3 minutes per side until crisp and golden.

6 Divide the fish cakes between four meal prep containers. Serve with lemon wedges, salad and sweet chilli sauce.

490
CALS

HONEY SOY GARLIC CHICKEN WITH RICE

PER SERVING | **490** CALS | **34G** PROTEIN | **21G** FAT | **41G** CARBS

prep
10 MINS

cook
45 MINS

FREEZE

SERVES 4

1 tbsp olive oil
3 tbsp dark soy sauce
2 tbsp honey
1 tbsp chopped
  fresh ginger
1 tbsp chopped
  fresh garlic
8 skinless, bone-in
  chicken thighs
2 tsp sesame seeds
160g rice
salt and pepper

This is delicious served with green beans and edamame.

1 Preheat the oven to 180°C fan.

2 In a bowl, combine the olive oil, soy sauce, honey, ginger and garlic, season with salt and pepper and mix thoroughly.

3 Put the chicken thighs in an ovenproof dish and pour over the sauce. Turn the thighs to coat in the mixture, then arrange them in the dish, fleshy side down to start with. Cover the dish with foil and cook for 20 minutes. Turn the thighs over so the fleshy side is facing up and sprinkle the tops with sesame seeds. Return to the oven, without the foil this time, for another 25 minutes until tender and browned.

4 While the chicken is cooking, cook the rice according to the packet instructions. Serve the chicken with rice, drizzling over any juices from the dish.

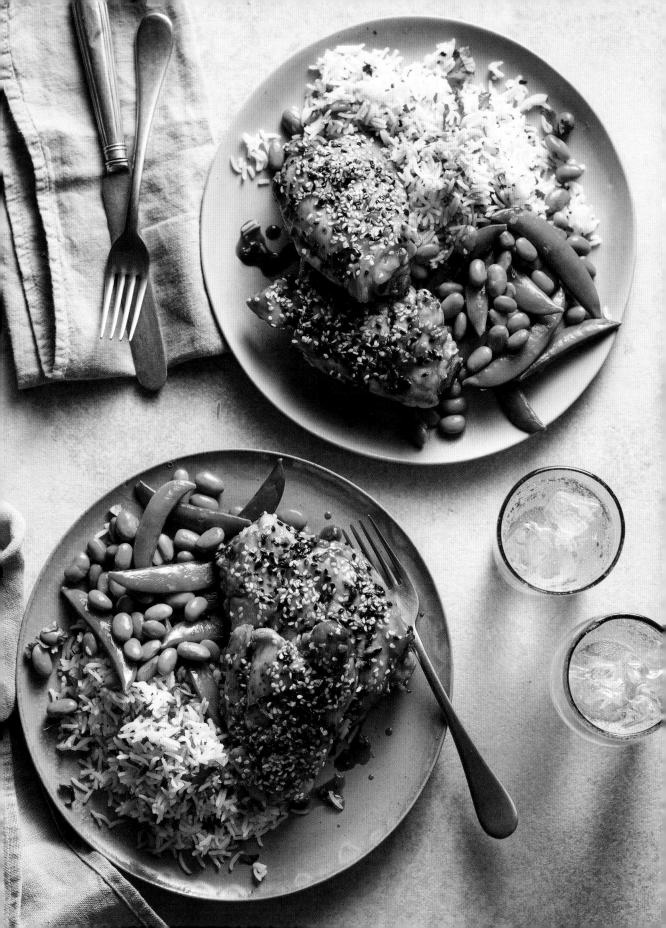

375
CALS

BUTTER CHICKEN

PER SERVING | **375** CALS | **39G** PROTEIN | **21G** FAT | **6G** CARBS

10 MINS   40 MINS   FREEZE

SERVES 6

1kg chicken breasts, diced
   into bite-sized pieces
low-calorie cooking
   oil spray
1 onion, finely chopped
3 tbsp butter
1 tbsp minced fresh garlic
1 tbsp minced fresh ginger
1 tbsp garam masala
1 tsp curry powder
¼ tsp cayenne pepper
   (if you like it a bit more
   spicy, you can add more)
1 x 400ml tin full-fat
   coconut milk
400g passata
salt and pepper
fresh coriander leaves,
   to garnish

A British curry house classic, made to be a little bit healthier.

1 Season the chicken with salt and pepper. Spray a large non-stick frying pan with cooking spray and add the chicken. Cook until the chicken is golden on the outside – it doesn't need to be cooked through.

2 Remove the chicken from the pan and set aside. Add the chopped onion and the butter and cook until the onion is golden and caramelized. Add the garlic, ginger and ground spices and cook together for about 1 minute, then add the coconut milk and the passata. Simmer with the lid off for about 20–25 minutes until the sauce is reduced and thickened.

3 Return the chicken to the pan and simmer for another 5 minutes until the chicken is cooked through. Season to taste with salt and pepper, then serve garnished with fresh coriander leaves, and with rice or naan breads on the side.

If you want to serve this with rice, allow for 50g of uncooked rice per person and each portion will be 497 calories.

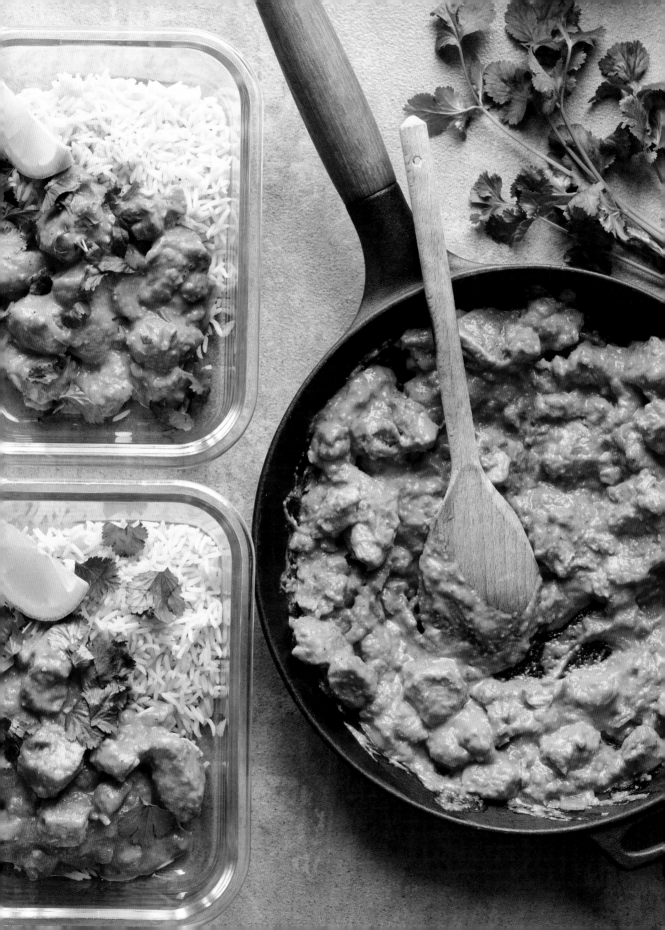

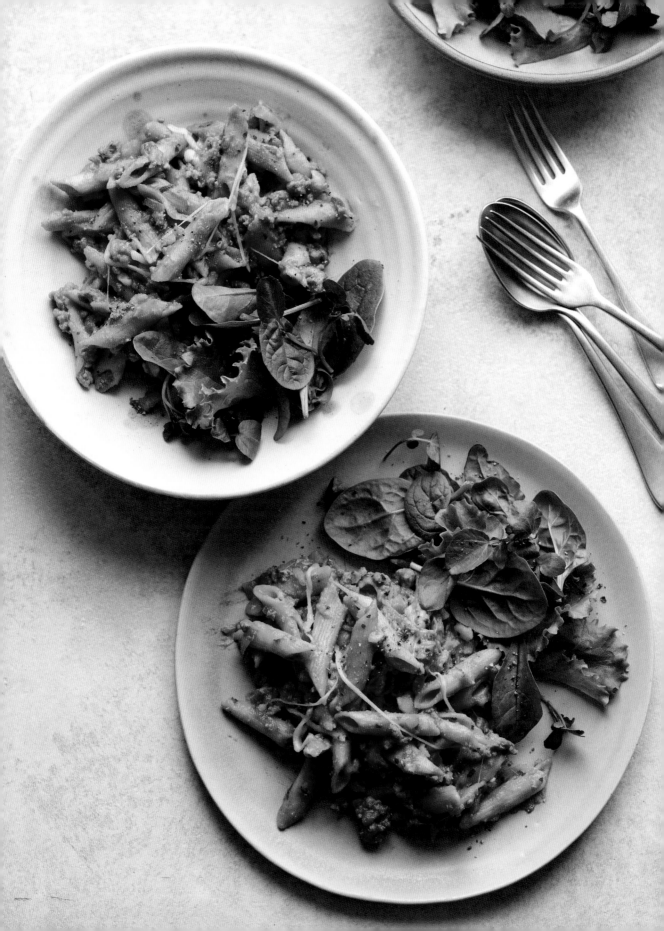

430
CALS

SLOW COOKER BAKED TURKEY PASTA

PER SERVING | **430** CALS | **40G** PROTEIN | **7G** FAT | **48G** CARBS

10 MINS   3.5–6.5 HOURS   FREEZE

SERVES 8

1 tbsp olive oil
750g lean turkey mince
1 large onion, finely diced
3 garlic cloves, minced
1kg passata
1 x 400g tin chopped
   tomatoes
2 tsp dried oregano
1 tsp dried basil
1 tsp salt
½ tsp pepper
1 chicken stock pot
500g wholewheat
   penne pasta
100g low-fat mozzarella
   cheese, grated
30g Parmesan cheese,
   grated, to serve
salad leaves, to serve
   (optional)

This is great for a meal prep day as we just chuck everything in the slow cooker and forget about it while we prep the rest of the week's meals.

1 Heat the oil in a large frying pan over medium-high heat. Add the mince and cook, stirring, for 3–4 minutes. Add the onion and garlic and continue cooking until the mince is cooked through.

2 Transfer the mince mixture to the slow cooker. Add the passata, chopped tomatoes, oregano and basil and season with salt and pepper. Dissolve the stock pot in 700ml boiling water, add this too and stir everything together.

3 Cover and cook for about 3 hours on HIGH or about 6 hours on LOW.

4 Add the pasta and continue cooking on the HIGH setting for about 20–40 minutes. Pasta cook times will vary, so after 20 minutes, begin checking it at 10-minute intervals to see if the pasta is done, stirring it once to make sure the pasta cooks evenly.

5 Stir half of the grated mozzarella into the slow cooker and sprinkle the remaining cheese on top. Cover and let stand for 5 minutes until the cheese on top is melted.

6 If using for meal prep, divide between the containers and allow to cool, then sprinkle the Parmesan cheese on top. No need to melt as you will do this when you reheat. Serve with salad leaves, if you like.

446
CALS

JERK COD WITH RICE 'N' PEAS

PER SERVING | **446** CALS | **34G** PROTEIN | **7G** FAT | **58G** CARBS

15 MINS   30 MINS   FREEZE

SERVES 4

2 tsp jerk seasoning
4 thick, skin-on cod fillets
   (about 140g each)
2 tsp olive oil

For the rice 'n' peas:
1 tbsp olive oil
1 large onion, finely diced
2 large garlic cloves,
   finely chopped
1 heaped tbsp fresh
   thyme leaves
200g long grain
   or basmati rice
1 Scotch bonnet chilli,
   halved
1 red pepper, finely diced
1 x 200g tin sweetcorn,
   drained
1 x 400g tin red kidney
   beans, drained and rinsed
4 spring onions, sliced
   and white and green
   parts separated
1 chicken stock pot
salt and pepper
lime wedges, to serve

This dish is inspired by Jamaican flavours, and makes a great meal prep, or an impressive dinner for friends.

1 First, get the rice and peas cooking. Put the oil in a large heavy-based saucepan on low–medium heat and add the onion. Cook for a good 6–7 minutes until the onion is very soft. Add the garlic and thyme and cook for another couple of minutes.

2 To the pan, add the rice, Scotch bonnet, red pepper, sweetcorn, kidney beans, spring onion whites, stock pot and 550ml water. Give everything a good stir and put a tight-fitting lid on the pan. Cook over medium heat for 12 minutes, then turn off the heat and let the rice finish cooking in the steam for another 10 minutes – don't take the lid off!

3 Meanwhile, prepare the fish. Sprinkle the jerk seasoning over the fillets and rub in so they are coated all over.

4 Heat the oil in a large non-stick frying pan over medium heat and add the fillets, skin-side down. Cook for 3–4 minutes until picking up some colour. Turn the fillets over with a fish slice and cook for another couple of minutes until golden on top and cooked through.

5 Once the rice is cooked, serve onto four plates or portion into meal prep containers and top with a fish fillet. Sprinkle with the spring onion greens to serve.

tip

Make sure you buy fish with the skin still on, as it will hold the fillets together during cooking.

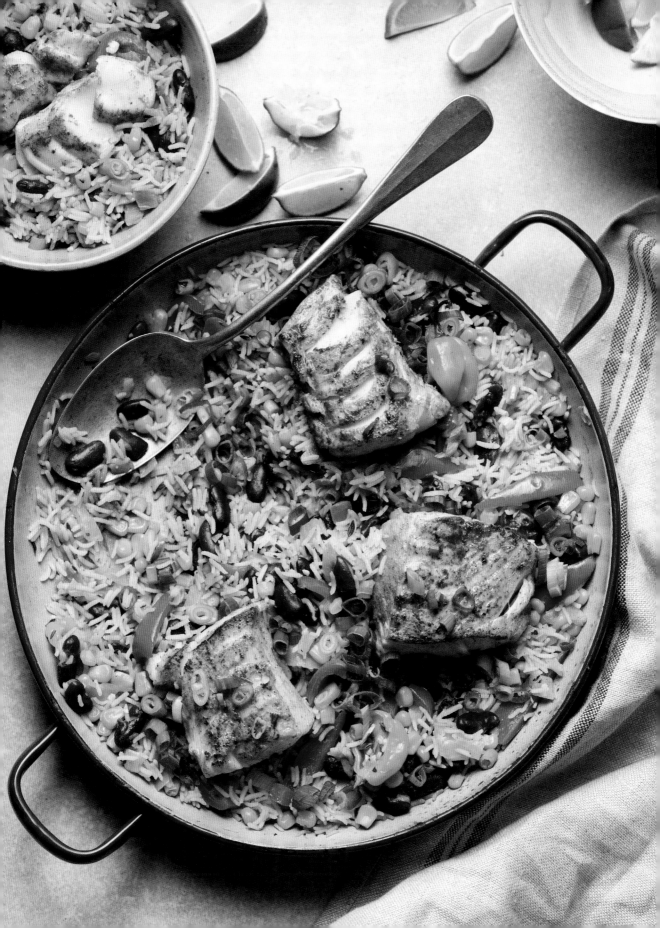

334 CALS

CHILLI CON QUINOA

PER SERVING | **334** CALS | **11G** PROTEIN | **8G** FAT | **74G** CARBS

10 MINS   35 MINS   FREEZE

SERVES 4

2 tbsp vegetable oil
1 onion, diced
3 carrots, peeled and diced
1 large red pepper,
    deseeded and diced
1 medium-large sweet
    potato, peeled and diced
2 garlic cloves, minced
2 tsp chilli powder
1 tsp ground cumin
½ tsp chipotle powder
    or smoked paprika
½ tsp sea salt, or more
    to taste
1 x 400g tin tomatoes
1 x 400g tin black beans,
    drained
400ml vegetable stock
90g uncooked quinoa
20g fresh coriander
    leaves, chopped
juice of ½ lime, or more
    to taste
soured cream (optional),
    to serve
wedge of lime (optional),
    to serve

*A fantastic meal prep that uses quinoa instead of rice.
The quinoa absorbs loads of flavour, making this a delicious
meal prep that doesn't need a side dish.*

1 Heat the oil in a large pan over medium heat. Add the onion
and cook, stirring occasionally, for about 5 minutes until it is
tender and some of the edges are brown. Add the carrots,
pepper and sweet potato and cook for another 5 minutes,
or until the vegetables are beginning to sweat.

2 Stir in garlic, chilli powder, cumin, chipotle powder and
the ½ tsp of salt. Cook, stirring occasionally, until the garlic
and spices begin to smell fragrant – about 2 minutes.

3 Pour in the tomatoes with their juices, then use a spoon to
scrape the bottom of the pot to remove any stuck browned
bits – there's flavour in these!

4 Stir in the beans, vegetable stock and quinoa. Bring the
chilli to a low simmer and cook, partially covered with a lid,
for 20 minutes, or until the quinoa is fully cooked. Taste and
season the chilli with additional salt if needed, then stir in
the coriander and lime juice.

5 Serve with soured cream and a wedge of lime.

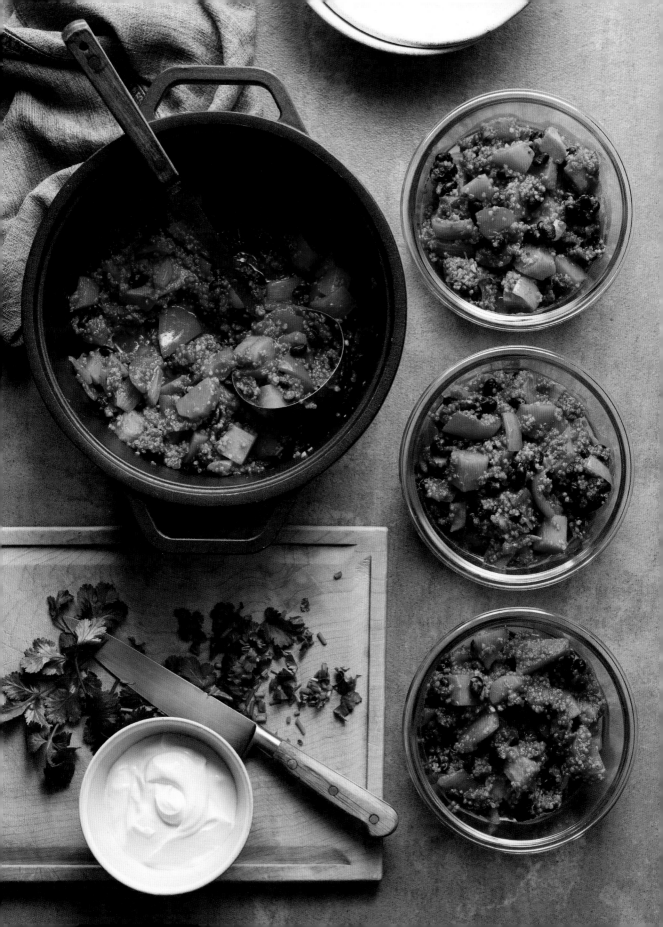

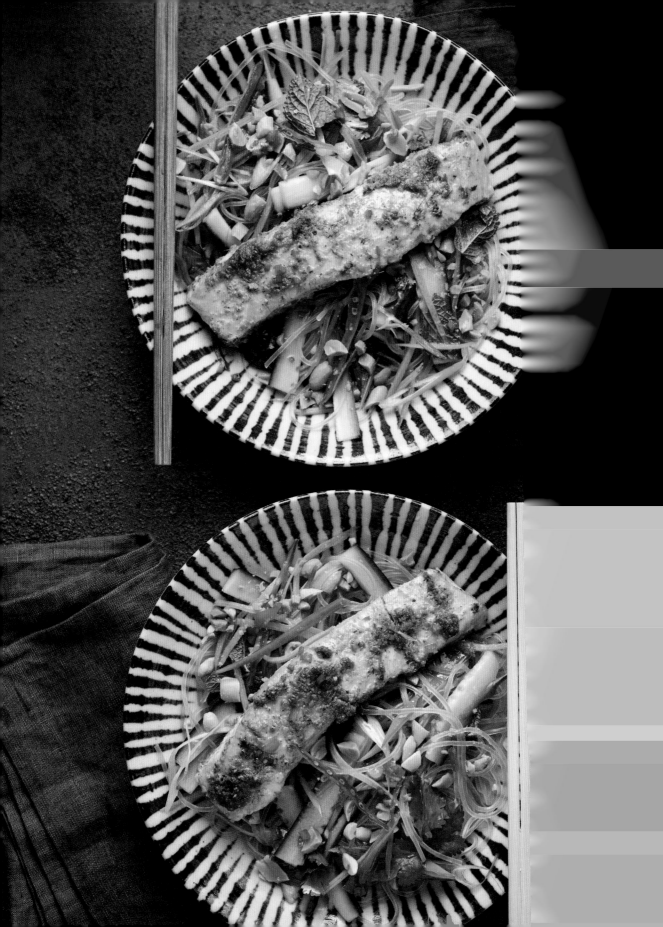

VIETNAMESE SALMON AND NOODLE SALAD

PER SERVING | **425** CALS | **31G** PROTEIN | **15G** FAT | **39G** CARBS

20 MINS +
MARINATING   20 MINS

SERVES 4

For the salmon and marinade:
1 stalk lemongrass,
    roughly chopped
2 garlic cloves,
    roughly chopped
1 red chilli, roughly chopped
2cm piece of fresh ginger,
    peeled and roughly
    chopped
a small handful of fresh
    coriander
zest and juice of 1 lime
1 tbsp nam pla (fish sauce)
4 salmon fillets

For the salad:
100g mangetout, julienned
100g beansprouts
1/2 cucumber, sliced
    into matchsticks
1 large carrot, peeled and
    chopped into matchsticks
6 spring onions, shredded
a large handful of fresh
    coriander leaves,
    roughly chopped
a small handful of fresh
    mint leaves, shredded
30g peanuts, roughly
    chopped
3 nests (150g) glass noodles

For the dressing:
juice of 3 limes
1 1/2 tbsp nam pla (fish sauce)
1 tbsp soft brown sugar
1 red chilli, finely chopped

Vietnamese food is usually quite hot, but you can vary the chilli in this to suit your own taste. If you want it hotter, use bird's eye chilli, and if milder, use a standard red chilli and remove the seeds.

1 Marinate the salmon in advance of cooking. Pop all the ingredients for the marinade in a blender and blitz until smoothish. Put the salmon in a baking dish and spread the marinade over the fillets to coat them completely. Cover with foil and place in the fridge to marinate for a few hours. Remove from the fridge and allow to come up to room temperature for 20 minutes before cooking.

2 To cook the salmon, preheat the oven to 180°C fan. Place the dish in the oven and bake for about 20 minutes, or until the salmon is just cooked through.

3 Meanwhile, prep your salad veg and put it all in a large serving bowl.

4 Put the noodles in a large bowl and cover with boiling water. Leave to cook as per the packet instructions (usually for 3–5 minutes, depending on brand), then drain. Tip them into the bowl with the salad veg.

5 Combine all the ingredients for the dressing and stir together, then pour this over the salad and toss to coat. If you are packing this as a meal prep, keep the dressing separate and toss it through the salad just before serving with the salmon.

492 CALS

TMPK BURGER (AKA FAKE BIG MAC)

PER SERVING | **492** CALS | **45G** PROTEIN | **15G** FAT | **43G** CARBS

prep 15 MINS   cook 5 MINS   FREEZE

SERVES 2

300g lean beef mince
low-calorie cooking
   oil spray
3 seeded brioche burger
   buns, sliced in half
¼ small onion, very
   finely chopped
2 leaves iceberg lettuce,
   shredded
2 low-fat processed
   cheese slices
2 gherkins (trust me), sliced
salt and pepper

For the sauce:
30g lighter than light mayo
15g American-style yellow
   mustard
¼ tsp sugar
½ tsp white vinegar

tip

*Don't be tempted to
overcook the beef patties.
Remember these will be
reheated. This will stop
them from becoming dry.*

My take on a fast food favourite.

1 Divide the meat into four even portions, and form each one into a thin patty, about the same diameter as the burger bun. Season the patties, then chill them for 1 hour.

2 Meanwhile, make the sauce by combining the mayonnaise, mustard, sugar and white vinegar. Season with salt and pepper, mix thoroughly and set aside.

3 Once the patties are chilled and firmed up, spritz a non-stick frying pan with a little cooking spray and fry them for a couple of minutes on each side until cooked through. Be careful not to overcook them or they will become dry.

4 Once the burgers are done, toast both the sides of each bun half in the same frying pan until lightly toasted.

5 To assemble your burger, place two of the bun bottoms on a worktop. If you are eating these right away, it's time for a spoonful of your special sauce spread over each base; if you're meal prepping these, divide the sauce between two separate sauce containers until you're ready to eat.

6 Sprinkle some of the finely chopped onion on top of the sauce on each burger, followed by a layer of shredded lettuce. Now add a meat patty to each base and top with a slice of cheese.

7 Here is where the third bun comes in. To make that classic centre bread layer of a Big Mac, use a half of the extra bun in each burger. On top of that, spread another spoonful of sauce and add a little more chopped onion and lettuce. Add some thinly sliced gherkins and the second meat patty. Pop the top of the bun on top to complete your creation.

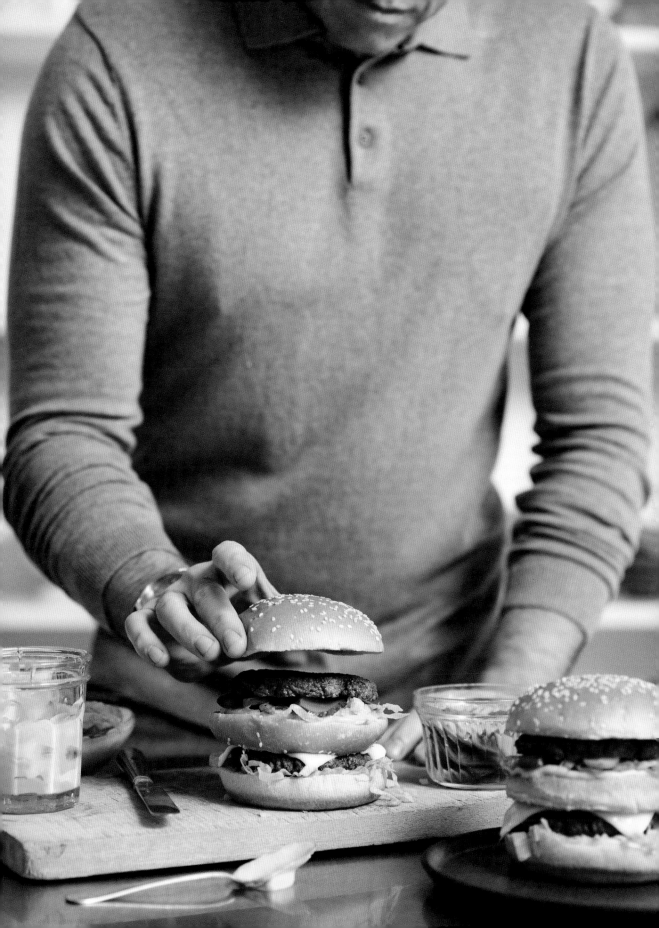

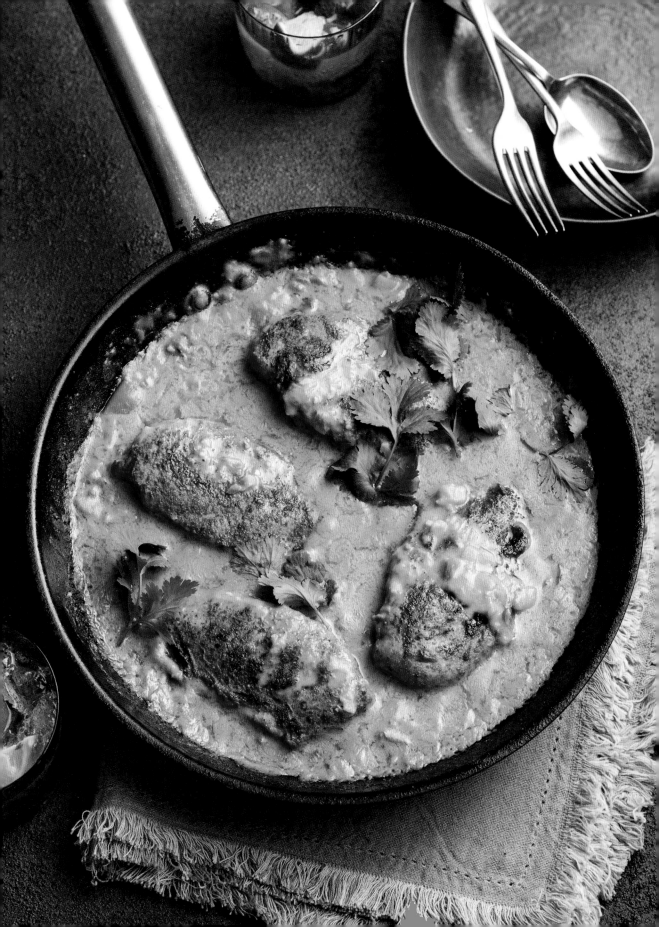

474
CALS

BRAZILIAN COCONUT CHICKEN CURRY AND RICE

PER SERVING | **474** CALS | **40G** PROTEIN | **17G** FAT | **39G** CARBS

prep 15 MINS   cook 30 MINS   FREEZE

SERVES 4

1 tsp ground turmeric
1 tsp ground cumin
1 tsp ground coriander
½ tsp garlic powder
1 tsp cayenne pepper
4 chicken breasts
    (about 150g each)
1 tbsp olive oil
1 onion, diced
1 garlic clove,
    finely chopped
1 red chilli, deseeded
    and finely sliced
1 chicken or vegetable
    stock cube
4 medium tomatoes, diced
grated zest of ½ lemon
    and a squeeze of juice
1 x 200ml tin light
    coconut milk
30g peanut butter
160g rice
salt and pepper
rice, to serve
fresh coriander or
    parsley, to garnish

The use of so many spices in this dish makes this meal prep irresistibly tasty. The flavours are just mouth-watering.

1 Preheat the oven to 180°C fan.

2 Combine all the spices in a bowl, then add the chicken breasts and turn them over to cover them completely in the spice.

3 Heat 1 tbsp of the olive oil in a casserole dish or ovenproof saucepan and fry the chicken breasts over medium heat until they are lightly browned all over. Remove from the pan and set aside.

4 Add the onion, garlic and chilli to the same pan and fry for 1–2 minutes before adding the stock cube, tomatoes, lemon juice and zest, coconut milk and peanut butter and mix through.

5 Return the chicken to the dish (along with any juices that leaked out) and cook on the hob for about 20 minutes, or until the chicken is cooked through and the sauce is reduced and thickened. Meanwhile, cook the rice according to the packet instructions.

6 Once it's had its 20 minutes, taste and season the curry, then serve with rice and garnish with fresh coriander or parsley.

Try adding some fresh chopped chillies for extra heat, for the brave.

444
CALS

MEXICAN-STYLE LASAGNE

PER SERVING | **444** CALS | **43G** PROTEIN | **18G** FAT | **25G** CARBS

20 MINS   50 MINS   FREEZE

SERVES 4

1 tbsp olive oil
2 peppers (any colour), chopped
1 green chilli, deseeded and finely chopped
1 red onion, diced
1 garlic clove, finely chopped
600g lean steak beef mince
1 x 400g tin chopped tomatoes
100g drained tinned sweetcorn
1 tsp Worcestershire sauce
2 tbsp fajita or Mexican seasoning, or more to taste
1 tbsp tomato purée
2 tortilla wraps
80g Cheddar cheese
salt and pepper

Tortilla wraps freeze really well, so feel free to freeze any you may have left.

This meal prep gives an interesting twist to a beloved classic.

1 Preheat the oven to 180°C fan.

2 Heat the oil in a large pan over medium heat, add the peppers, chilli, onion and garlic and cook for a few minutes until the veg is softening. Add the mince and cook, stirring frequently, until browned.

3 Add the chopped tomatoes to the pan, then fill the empty can about one-third full with water. Swill it around to catch all the remaining tomato juice and tip that into the pan too. Add the sweetcorn, Worcestershire sauce, Mexican seasoning and tomato purée to the pan and season with salt and pepper. Reduce the heat to low and simmer for 10–15 minutes, until the sauce is reduced and thickened.

4 When everything is cooked, spread one-third of the meat mixture over the base of an ovenproof dish. Using a tortilla as you would lasagne sheets, layer it over the meat, ripping it up if needed to cover the meat. Add another layer of mince, followed by the other tortilla, then add a final layer of mince. Top the lasagne with grated cheese and place in the oven for 25 minutes, until the cheese is golden brown.

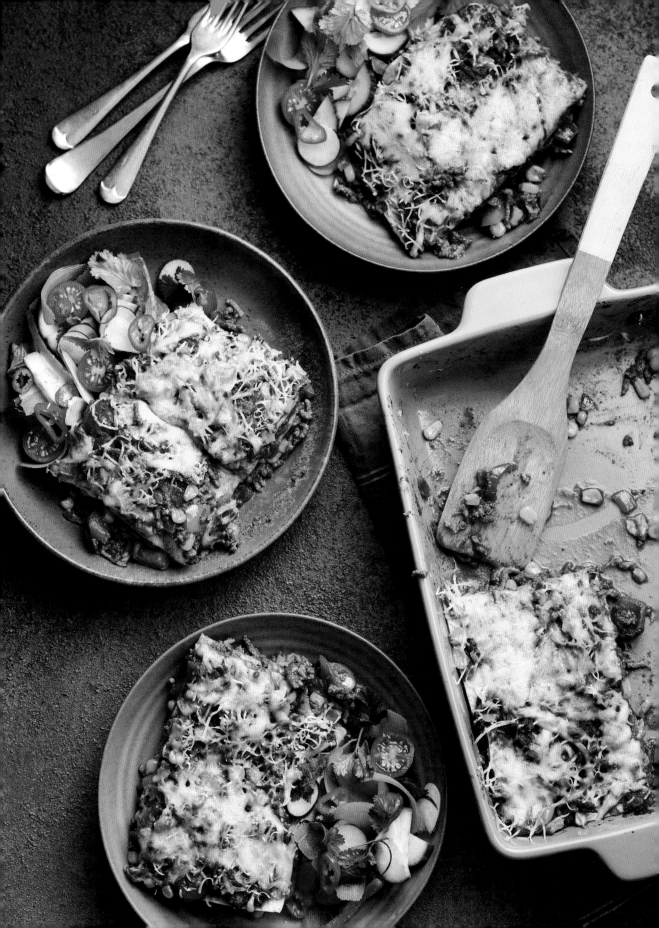

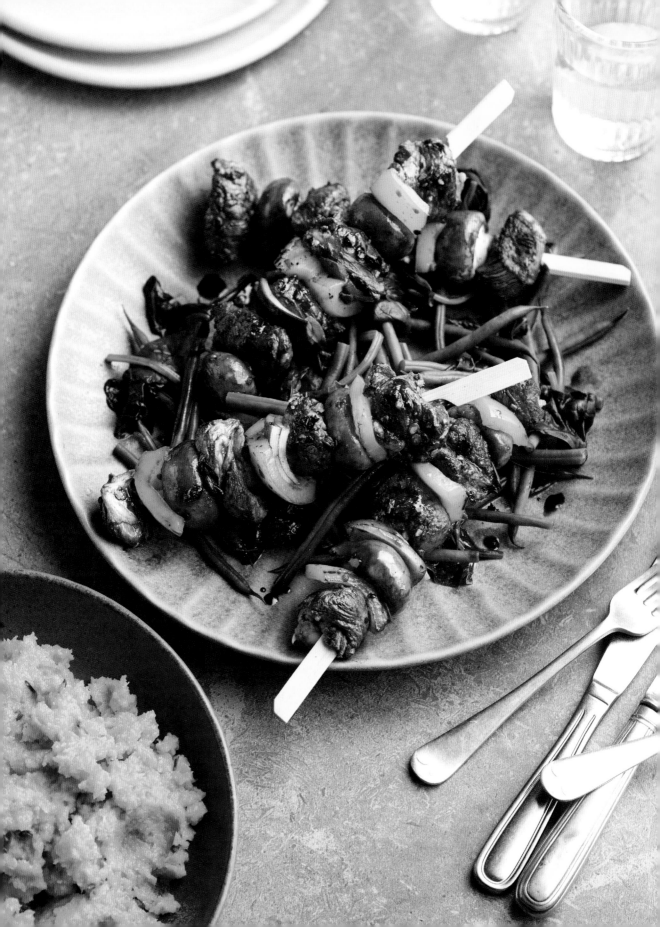

LAMB KEBABS WITH ROSEMARY AND RED WINE CHILLI GLAZE

PER SERVING | **226** CALS | **19G** PROTEIN | **7G** FAT | **12G** CARBS

20 MINS + MARINATING 30 MINS FREEZE

SERVES 4

187ml red wine
   (one mini bottle)
2 large garlic cloves,
   finely chopped
1 tbsp chopped fresh
   rosemary
350g lean lamb
   (cut into 16 cubes)
3 tbsp honey
2 tsp ancho chilli flakes
1 small red onion,
   cut into squares
1 yellow pepper,
   chopped into squares
16 smallish mushrooms
a drizzle of oil,
   for the griddle
salt and pepper
Root mash (see page 181)
   and green beans, or
   flatbreads, to serve

Lamb, peppers and chilli are just meant to go together. These are great cooked on a barbecue or in a cast iron griddle pan.

1 In a glass or ceramic bowl, mix together the wine, garlic and rosemary and season well with salt and pepper. Add the lamb chunks and leave to marinate in the fridge for a few hours.

2 Once the lamb has marinated, tip the marinade into a saucepan and stir in the honey and chilli flakes. Set the pan over a medium heat and cook, stirring regularly, for 20 minutes or so until it has reduced to a sticky glaze. Season well with salt and pepper.

3 Meanwhile, thread the lamb chunks onto eight skewers, alternating with chunks of the onion and pepper and the mushrooms. Preheat a griddle pan to medium-high heat.

4 Cook the skewers on the griddle, drizzling it with a tiny bit of oil first and cooking in two batches if necessary, for about 10 minutes, turning every 2–3 minutes to cook each side. Towards the end of cooking, liberally brush on the glaze and allow the kebabs to char slightly, but make sure the lamb is still pink in the middle.

5 Serve the skewers with the root mash and green beans or with flatbreads.

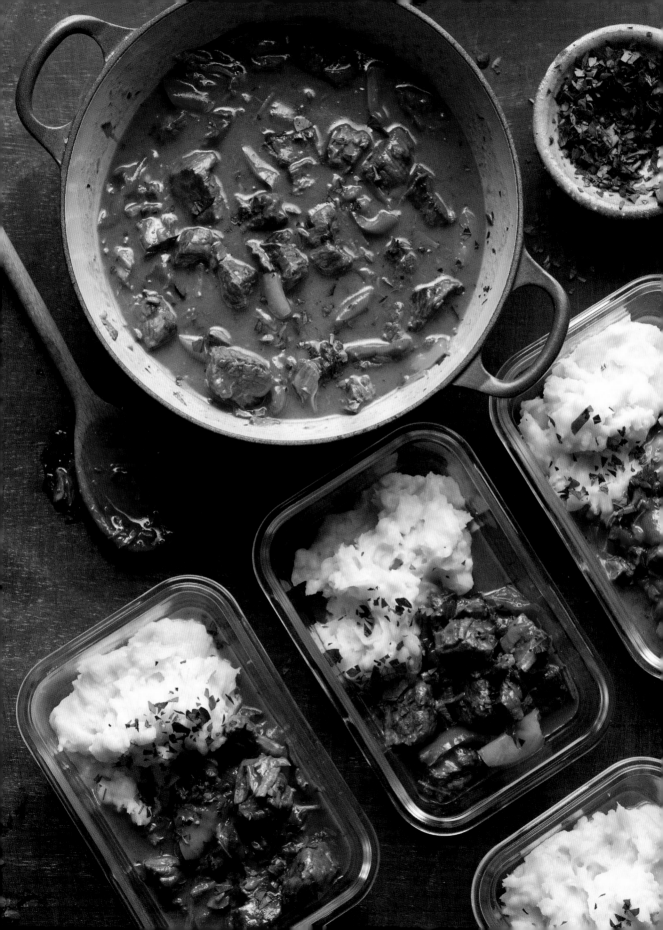

363
CALS

SLOW COOKER BEEF AND PEPPERS

PER SERVING | **363** CALS | **49G** PROTEIN | **14G** FAT | **9G** CARBS

prep
10 MINS

cook
3–7 HOURS

FREEZE

SERVES 8

2 tbsp olive oil
1.5kg lean braising steak, diced
1 onion, sliced
2 red peppers, chopped into 2.5cm cubes
2 yellow peppers, chopped into 2.5cm cubes
1 tbsp garlic granules
1 tsp salt
2 tsp pepper
600ml hot beef stock
2–3 tbsp sriracha hot sauce (to taste)
2 tsp Worcestershire sauce
3 tbsp cornflour
chopped fresh parsley, to sprinkle

We also love this served with bulghur wheat.

A hearty warming dish the whole family is sure to love. Try serving with potato mash as they make such a good combo.

1 In a large frying pan, heat the oil over a high heat and fry the meat for just a few minutes until you start to see some colour. You may want to do this in batches, dividing the oil between the batches, so that the pan isn't overcrowded and the meat browns quickly. Remove the meat from the pan, leaving the fat in the pan, turn down the heat to medium–low and add the onion. Cook for a few minutes until softened, then add to the slow cooker along with your chopped peppers, garlic granules, salt and pepper.

2 Mix the beef stock with the sriracha and Worcestershire sauce and pour over the peppers and beef. Cook on HIGH for 3–4 hours or on LOW for 6–7 hours.

3 Two hours before the end of cooking on LOW and 1 hour before the end on HIGH, mix the cornflour with a splash of water to a smooth paste. Tip it into the slow cooker and mix in well. Replace the lid to let it finish cooking and thicken the sauce a little.

4 Once cooked and it's all nice and thick, separate the stew into meal prep containers. To serve, sprinkle with the parsley and serve with the accompanying carb of your choice.

427
CALS

HOMEMADE DONER KEBAB

PER SERVING | **427** CALS | **37G** PROTEIN | **11G** FAT | **43G** CARBS

prep 20 MINS *cook* 45 MINS FREEZE

SERVES 3

200g lamb mince (lowest
   % fat you can find)
200g low-fat beef mince
1 tsp smoked paprika
1 tsp garlic granules
1 tsp oregano
1 tsp onion salt
1 tsp ground cumin
1 tsp ground coriander
20g fresh parsley or
   coriander, finely chopped
salt and pepper

For the sauce:
3 tbsp fat-free plain yogurt
juice of ¼ lemon
1 garlic clove, minced
30g cucumber, grated
1 tbsp chopped fresh
   coriander or parsley

To serve:
3 flatbreads (75g each)
a little shredded red
   or white cabbage
a few slices of white onion
a few slices of cucumber
1 large tomato, sliced

tip

*To reheat the doner meat,
try frying thin strips in
a little vegetable oil to
bring it back to life.*

An amazing Friday night fake-away!

1 Preheat the oven to 180°C fan.

2 Firstly, rinse and wash an empty 400g tin. I use an old
baked bean tin, but you can use any you like. Remove the
lid if it's still attached to the top.

3 In a mixing bowl, combine the lamb and beef mince, spices
and parsley or coriander, and season with salt and pepper.
Mix together well with your hands.

4 Pack the meat mixture into the tin and press down firmly.
Put the tin in an ovenproof dish or glass meal prep container
and add a little water to the bottom so it comes about 2cm
up the sides of the tin. Cover the top of the tin with a little
tin foil. Cook in the preheated oven for 40 minutes, or until
cooked throughout.

5 Whilst the meat is cooking, make the sauce. Put the yogurt,
lemon juice, garlic, cucumber and herbs in a small bowl and
season with salt and pepper. Mix and set aside.

6 Once cooked, leave the meat to rest in the tin for 5 minutes,
then remove from the tin in one piece, remembering it will still
be quite hot. You may have to turn the tin over and use a tin
opener to remove the bottom in order to push the meat out.

7 Heat a frying pan over a high heat and place the meat
in. Brown the outside of the meat on all sides until charred.
Or you could use a chef's blow torch to char the outside.

8 Slice thin strips off the side of the 'doner' and serve
in flatbreads, topped with the sauce and salad.

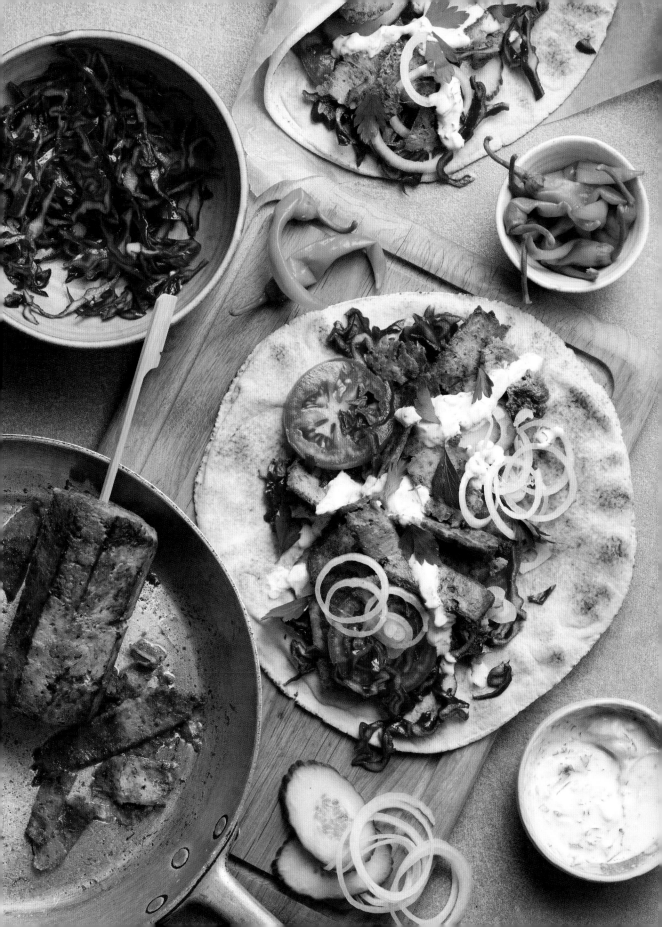

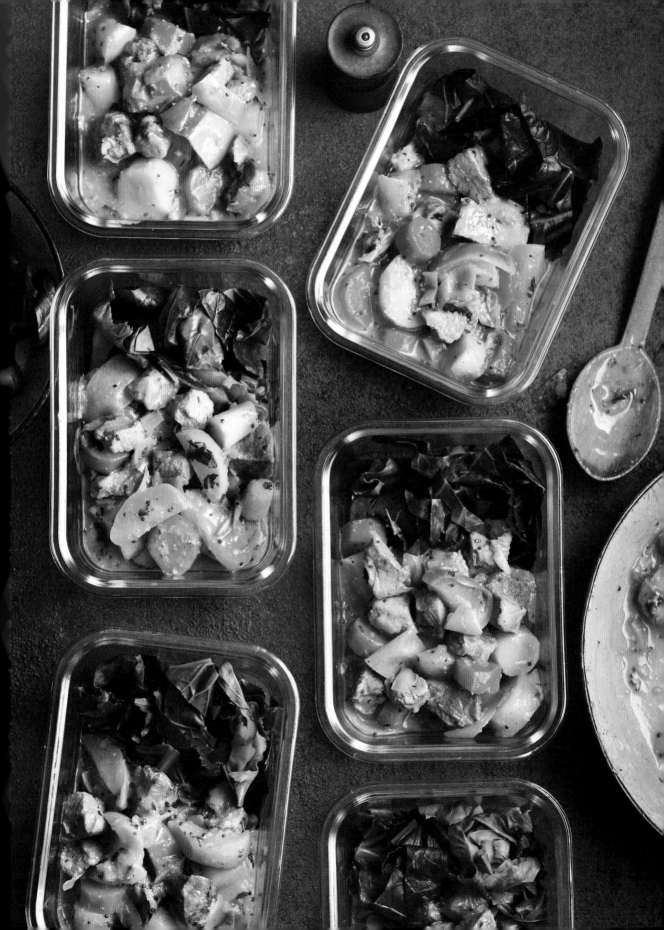

425
CALS

SLOW COOKER PORK WITH APPLES AND CIDER

PER SERVING | **425** CALS | **37G** PROTEIN | **10G** FAT | **37G** CARBS

prep
15 MINS

cook
4–8 HOURS

FREEZE

SERVES 6

1 tbsp olive oil
900g extra-lean diced pork
1 large onion, chopped into large dice
2 leeks, cut into slim slices
600g parsnips, peeled and cut into large chunks
600g carrots, peeled and chopped into large chunks
500ml cider
1 chicken stock pot
2 tsp wholegrain mustard
a small bunch of fresh thyme sprigs
3 eating apples
3 tbsp cornflour
salt and pepper
a handful of fresh parsley, chopped, to serve (optional)

An amazingly comforting meal prep that just gets better the longer you cook it.

1 Start by browning the pork. Add half of the oil to a large non-stick frying pan over high heat and cook half of the pork until browned all over. Add to the slow cooker, then use the remaining oil to brown the other half of the meat and add that to the slow cooker too.

2 Add the onion, leeks, parsnips, carrots and cider to the pot. Dissolve the stock pot and mustard in 400ml boiling water from the kettle and add that too, then chuck in the thyme sprigs and give it all a good stir. Cook on HIGH for 3 hours or on LOW for 6 hours.

3 Once the stew has had this time, put the cornflour in a small bowl or mug with a splash of water and mix it to a runny paste. Stir this into the stew.

4 Peel and core the apples and slice each of them into six wedges, then add these to the slow cooker too. Give everything a good stir then cook for a final 1 hour on HIGH or 2 hours on LOW. Season to taste with salt and pepper and extract the thyme stalks. Serve straight away or portion into meal prep containers for freezing or enjoying later in the week. Sprinkle with a little parsley to serve, if you like.

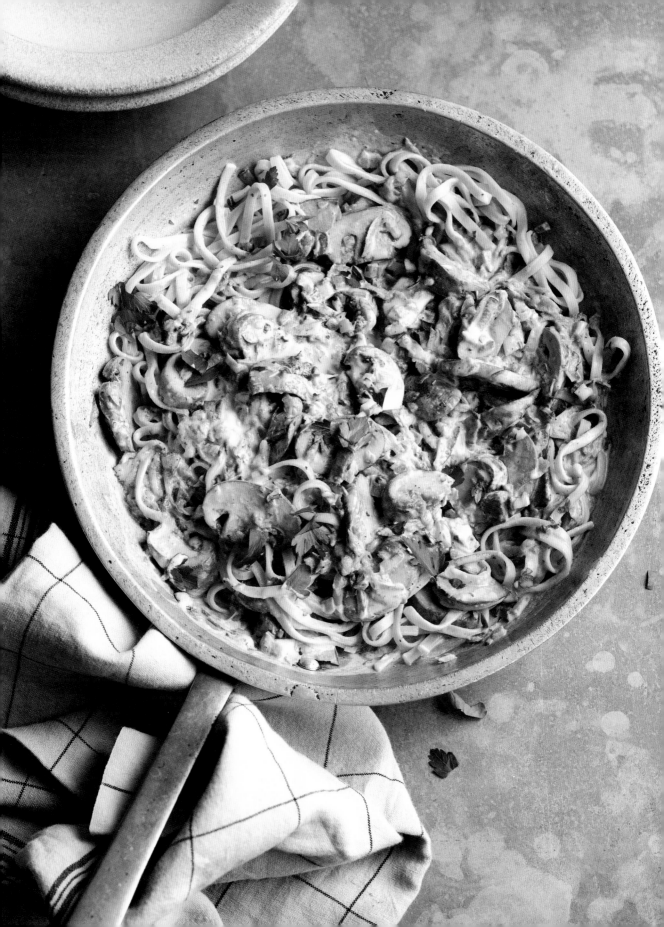

MUSHROOM AND COURGETTE STROGANOFF

PER SERVING | **435** CALS | **14G** PROTEIN | **15G** FAT | **58G** CARBS

15 MINS   25 MINS

SERVES 4

2 tbsp olive oil
1 onion, finely diced
1 tsp dried thyme
3 garlic cloves, finely
   chopped
500g mushrooms, sliced
1 courgette, grated
1 mushroom or vegetable
   stock pot
1 tsp grainy or Dijon
   mustard
80g crème fraîche
a small handful of fresh
   flatleaf parsley, chopped
salt and pepper
300g tagliatelle or
   pappardelle pasta,
   to serve

The addition of courgette here makes this a bit lighter and also allows you to shoehorn a bit more veg into your meal. Use whichever mushrooms take your fancy - packs of exotic varieties make it more interesting, but you can also use a basic chestnut variety. This is also great served with rice.

1 Heat the oil in a large sauté pan and add the onion. Cook over a low heat for 5-6 minutes until well softened. Add the thyme, garlic and mushrooms and increase the heat to medium. Cook for a few minutes until the mushrooms are softened and wilted down. Add the courgette to the pan and cook for another few minutes, until all the veg are really starting to soften.

2 Dissolve the stock pot in 200ml boiling water, then add it to the pan. Stir in the mustard and cook for a good 10 minutes, until everything is well cooked and the sauce is beginning to reduce down. Stir in the crème fraîche, then taste and season. Cook for a couple of minutes to get it back up to temperature, then stir in the parsley and either serve straight away with pasta, or pack it all into a meal prep container and store in the fridge to be enjoyed later in the week.

446 CALS

ROASTED VEGETABLE LASAGNE

PER SERVING | **446** CALS | **19G** PROTEIN | **15G** FAT | **56G** CARBS

prep 25 MINS   *cook* 1 HOUR   FREEZE

SERVES 6

1 large red onion, half chopped into wedges and the other half finely diced

2 peppers (any colour you wish), deseeded and cut into 2.5cm (1in) pieces

1 large yellow or green courgette

450g sweet potato or butternut squash flesh, cut into 2cm cubes

3 tbsp olive oil

2 garlic cloves, minced

2 x 400g tins chopped tomatoes

2 tsp dried oregano

1 vegetable stock cube

8–10 lasagne sheets (fresh or dried)

60g low-fat Cheddar cheese

salt and pepper

For the white sauce:
60g low-fat margarine
60g plain flour
600ml semi-skimmed milk
80g low-fat Cheddar cheese

1 Preheat the oven to 190°C fan. Put the onion wedges, peppers, courgette and sweet potato or butternut on a baking tray (use a second tray if it's looking too cramped). Drizzle over 2 tbsp of the olive oil and season with salt and pepper, then roast for 20–25 minutes, or until soft and caramelizing slightly.

2 Meanwhile, add the remaining oil to a large frying pan and sauté the diced onion for 3–4 minutes. Add the garlic, tomatoes and oregano and mix together. Quarter fill both tomato tins with water and swill out the tins, pouring the tomatoey water into the pan. Add the stock cube and leave to simmer, stirring occasionally, for 15 minutes or until the mixture has thickened. Once thickened, stir in the roasted vegetables.

3 For the white sauce, melt the margarine in a saucepan over a low heat. Add the flour and cook for 1–2 minutes. Add the milk, a little at a time, while continually whisking to get rid of any lumps. Cook the sauce for a good 5–10 minutes until thickened, stirring frequently, then turn off the heat and add the cheese. Keep stirring until the cheese has melted and you have a nice smooth consistency, then season to taste.

4 Spoon a layer of the vegetable mixture into a large baking dish – you want to use about half of the vegetable mix. Cover with a single layer of the lasagne sheets. Don't worry if you have to break some up to fit around the edge. Add half of the white sauce to the dish, followed by another layer of the veg mix, using it all up this time. Lay down one more layer of lasagne sheets and cover with the remaining white sauce. Finish by sprinkling the grated cheese over the top of the lasagne.

5 Bake for 30 minutes, or until the cheese is brown and bubbling. Eat whatever portions you want to enjoy now, then let the rest cool before slicing into portions and transferring to containers to chill and reheat later.

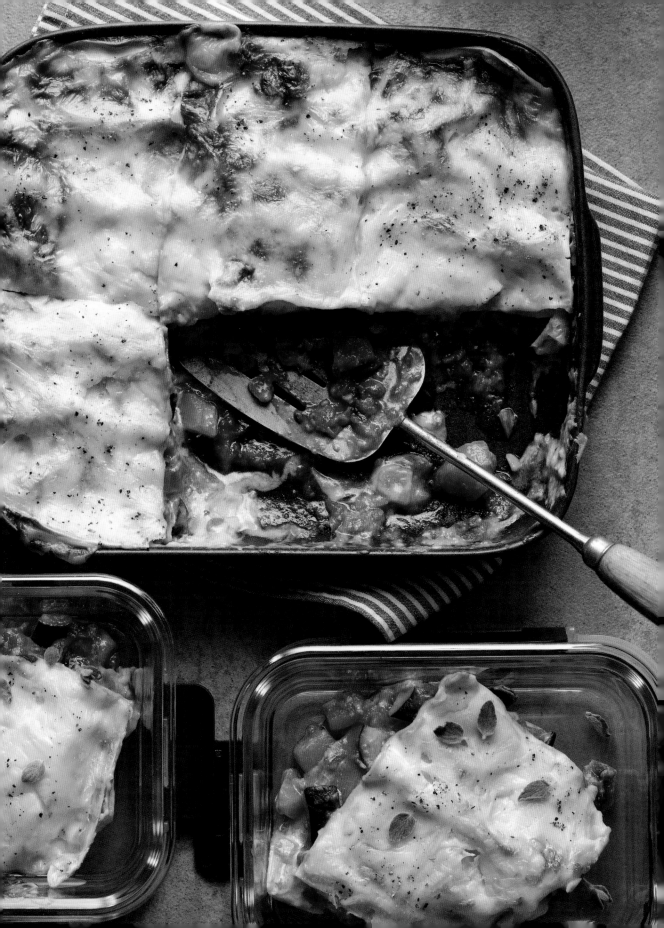

499
CALS

FISH FINGERS, PEAS AND MASH

PER SERVING | **499** CALS | **36G** PROTEIN | **6G** FAT | **71G** CARBS

20 MINS + CHILLING   30 MINS   FREEZE

SERVES 4

500g thick cod loin fillets
½ tsp salt
1kg mashing potatoes
40g plain flour
2 eggs, beaten
80g golden breadcrumbs
20g low-fat margarine
50ml skimmed milk
240g garden peas
salt and pepper
lemon wedges, to serve

Why not let the kids help out in the kitchen? A great meal prep to get the kids interested in cooking.

1 Cut the cod into fish finger-sized strips, then sprinkle with the ½ tsp salt. Cover and set aside in the fridge for 30 minutes; this will help firm up the fish fingers.

2 Meanwhile, preheat the oven to 200°C fan and lightly grease a baking tray.

3 Peel and slice the potatoes into large chunks. Drop into a pan of salted boiling water and cook for 20–25 minutes until very soft.

4 Put the flour in a shallow bowl, the eggs in a second bowl and the breadcrumbs in a third. One at a time, coat each piece of cod first in the flour, then in the egg, then roll in the breadcrumbs so each piece is evenly coated. Place the fish fingers on the prepared baking tray and bake for 15–20 minutes until crisp and golden and cooked throughout.

5 Once the potatoes are cooked, drain them and let them steam dry in the colander for a minute. Tip back into the hot pan and add the margarine, milk and plenty of seasoning. Mash until smooth.

6 Cook the peas either in the microwave or in a pan of boiling water for 3 minutes, then drain.

7 Serve the fish fingers with the mash, peas and lemon wedges, or pop it all into meal prep containers to enjoy later in the week.

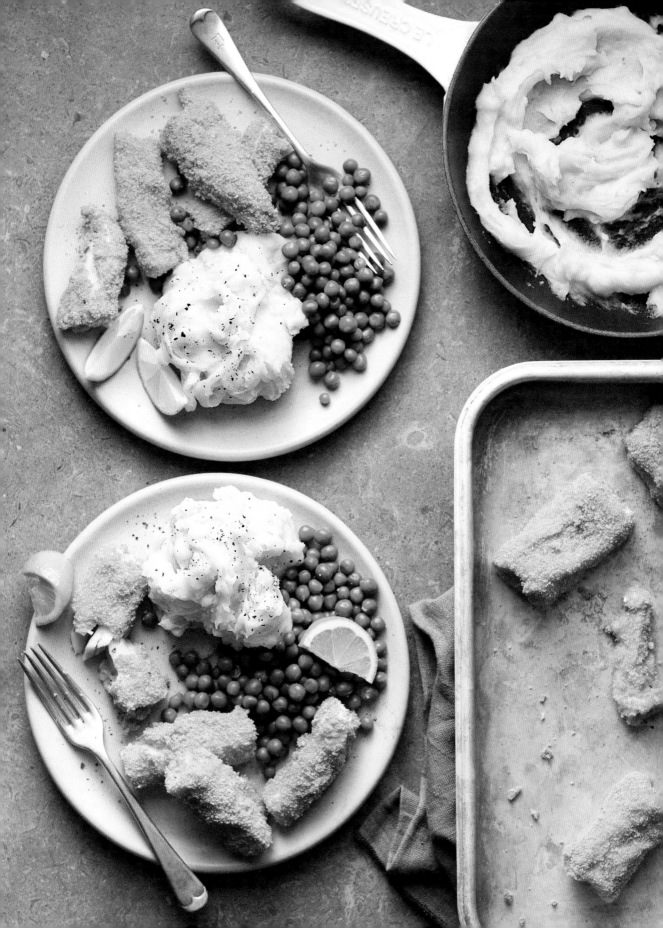

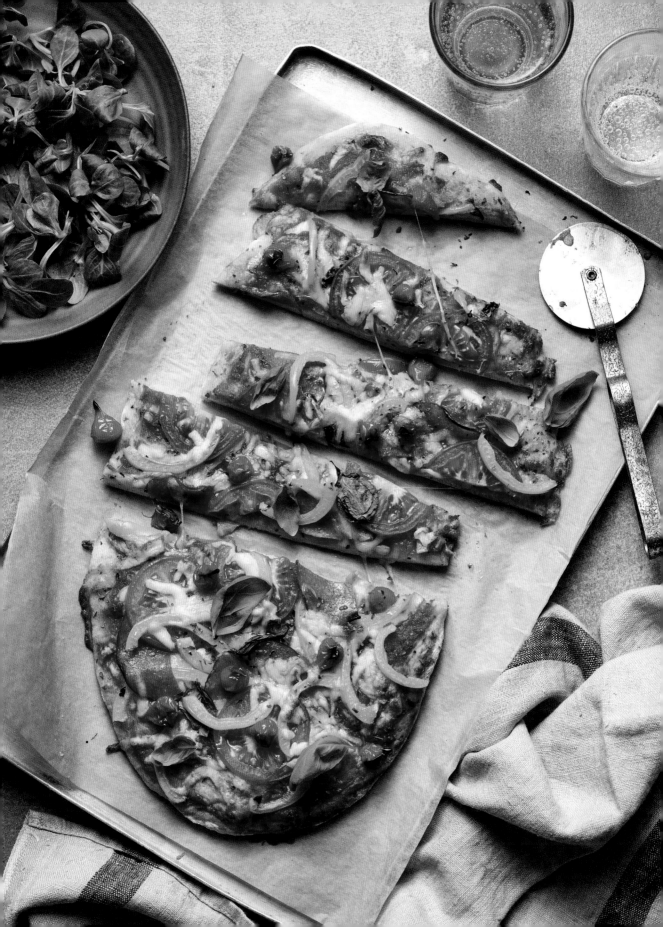

489 CALS

FAKE-AWAY FRIDAY NIGHT PIZZA

PER SERVING | **489** CALS | **23G** PROTEIN | **9G** FAT | **75G** CARBS

prep 30 MINS + PROVING   **cook** 15 MINS   **FREEZE**

SERVES 2

For the dough:
175g strong white
   bread flour
½ x 7g sachet (or 1 tsp)
   of dried yeast
salt and pepper

For the toppings:
1 large tomato, sliced
60g sliced yellow pepper
125g passata
15g pepperoni slices,
   halved
100g low-fat
   mozzarella cheese
1 tsp dried oregano
15g fresh basil leaves
25g sweety drop red
   peppers

*For an extra treat you
can add extra cheese,
if you like, but just
remember to add
the calories.*

*Pizzas are notoriously high in calories and salt. This is a great
alternative to save on calories and money as takeaways can
be expensive.*

1 Preheat the oven to its highest temperature, set a shelf
at the top of the oven and put a pizza stone or heavy baking
tray on the top shelf to heat up as the oven heats.

2 To make the dough, put the flour, yeast and 110ml warm
water in a large bowl with salt and pepper and knead for
2–3 minutes. Alternatively, you can use a stand mixer fitted
with a dough hook.

3 Once you have a smooth, stretchy dough, cover with a tea
towel dampened with warm water and leave to prove until
doubled in size.

4 While the dough proves, prep the toppings. Chop up the
tomato and pepper and organize all your toppings on the side,
making sure to weigh them all.

5 Uncover the pizza dough and roll it out into a large circle or
oval on some baking paper (make sure it will fit on your pizza
stone), making it thicker at the edges. Spread with the passata,
going almost to the edges, then sprinkle with your toppings.

6 Carefully remove the pizza stone from the oven and slide
the pizza onto it, still on its baking paper. Return the stone
to the top shelf, Reduce the heat to 180°C fan and cook for
12 minutes until the cheese is melted and the base is crisp.

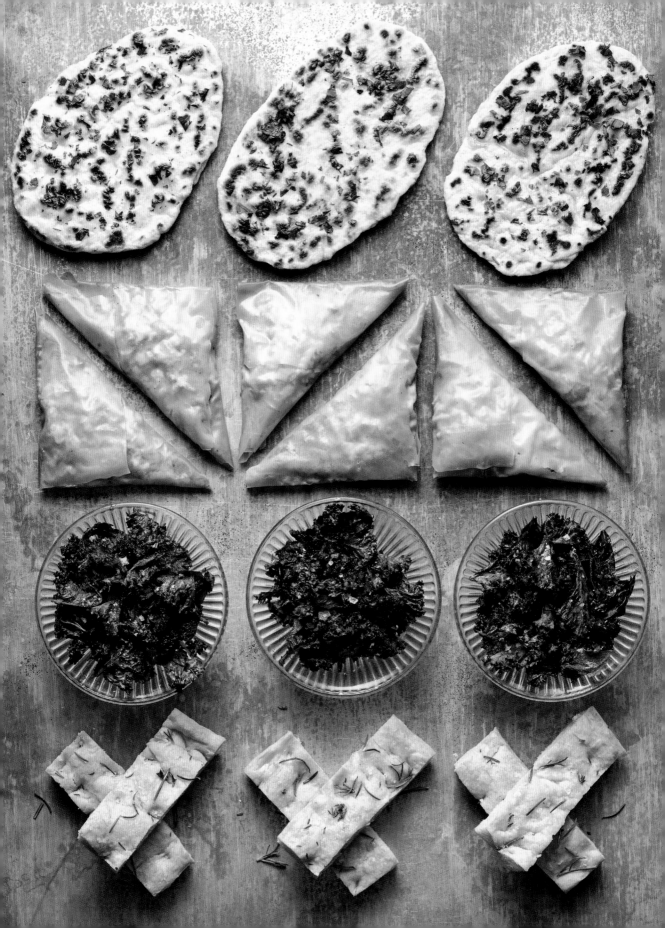

SNACKS AND SIDES

TOASTY TRAIL MIXES

These are great for taking in little containers on the go. Full of toasty flavours and sweet treats, they will give you an energy boost when you're flagging.

MOCHA PECAN PICK-ME-UP

PER SERVING | 3G PROTEIN | 8G FAT | 22G CARBS

172 CALS | prep 5 MINS | cook 5 MINS

MAKES 6 PORTIONS

50g pecan nuts
80g buckwheat groats
60g raisins
10g coffee beans
40g dark chocolate chunks
a pinch of salt

1 Preheat the oven to 180°C fan.

2 Sprinkle the pecans and the buckwheat groats onto a baking tray and toast in the oven for 5 minutes. Let cool completely (or they will melt the chocolate).

3 Once cool, combine the toasted pecans and buckwheat with all the remaining ingredients. Divide between six small containers, ready to take with you on the go.

BANANA BERRY BRAN

PER SERVING | 3G PROTEIN | 10G FAT | 25G CARBS

208 CALS | prep 5 MINS | cook 6 MINS

MAKES 6 PORTIONS

30g pumpkin seeds
30g coconut flakes
50g dried banana chips
60g bran flakes
75g dried berries (a mix of blueberries, cranberries, cherries, etc.)
30g white chocolate chips
a pinch of salt

1 Preheat the oven to 180°C fan.

2 Sprinkle the pumpkin seeds onto a baking tray and toast in the oven for 3 minutes. Add the coconut flakes to the tray and return the tray to the oven for another 2–3 minutes, or until the coconut is light golden. Let cool completely (or they will melt the chocolate).

3 Once cool, combine the toasted pumpkin seeds and coconut flakes with all the remaining ingredients. Divide between six small containers, ready to take with you on the go.

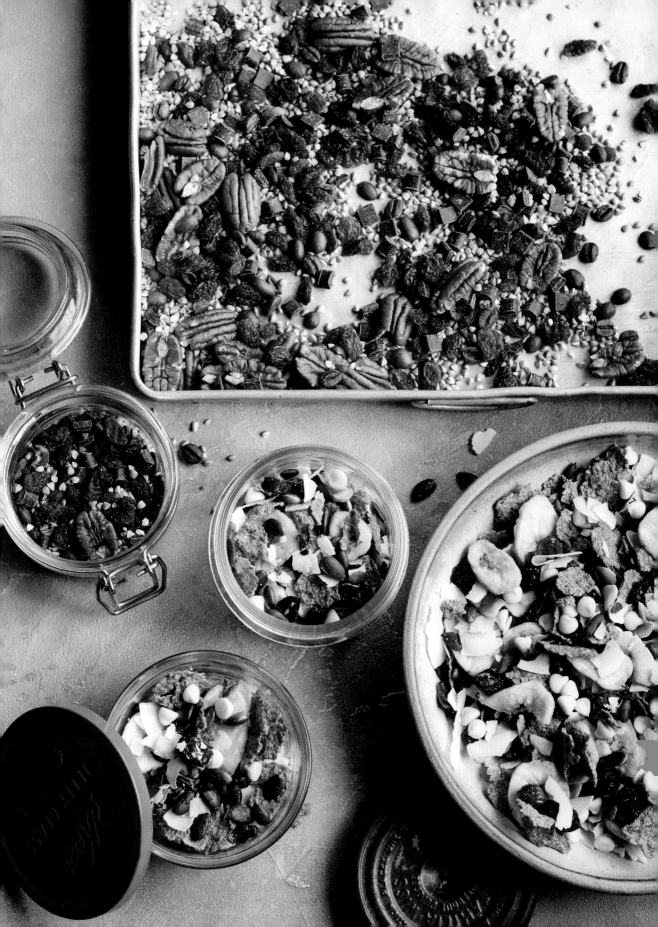

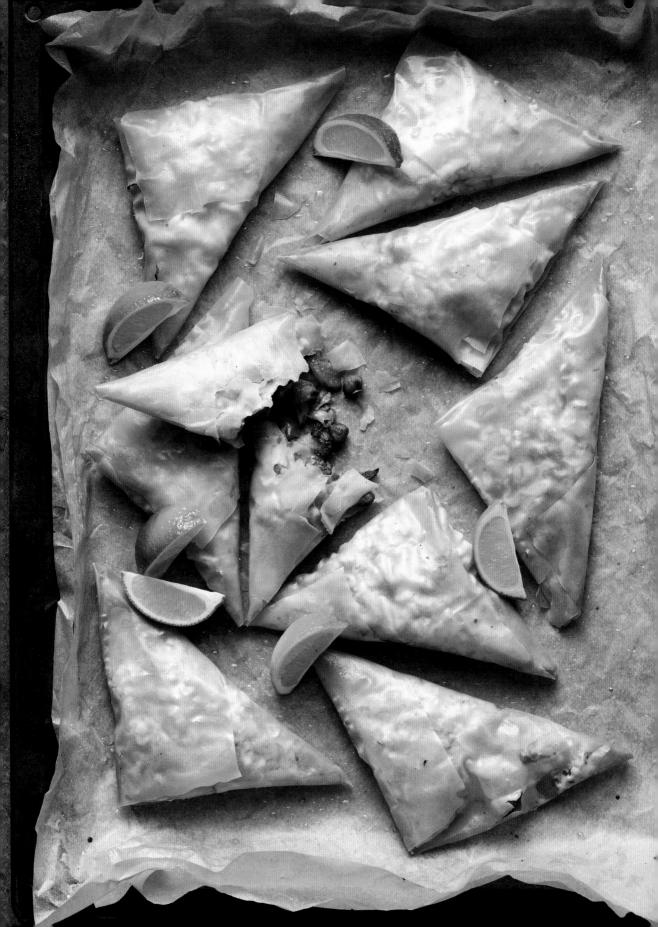

CURRIED VEG AND PANEER SAMOSAS

PER SAMOSA | 198 CALS | 9G PROTEIN | 7G FAT | 22G CARBS

prep **25 MINS**   cook **1 HOUR 5 MINS**   **FREEZE**

MAKES 12

3 red peppers, deseeded and chopped into 2.5cm chunks
350g very small cauliflower florets
1 large red onion, chopped into slim wedges
2 tbsp olive oil
1 x 400g tin chickpeas, drained
175g paneer cheese, chopped into 1cm cubes
3 tbsp rogan josh curry paste
5 tbsp passata
6 large sheets filo pastry
1 tbsp butter, melted
salt

Delicious pockets of cheese and roasted veggies, all flavoured with Indian spices.

1 Preheat the oven to 180°C fan.

2 Put the veg in a large bowl and drizzle over the olive oil. Sprinkle with a good pinch of salt and toss so everything is coated in oil. Tip onto a large baking tray and pop in the oven to roast for 30 minutes, stirring halfway through, until soft and beginning to turn brown.

3 When the 30 minutes are up, add the chickpeas and paneer to the tray, along with the curry paste. Stir so everything is well coated, then return to the oven for a final 10 minutes. Once out of the oven, stir the passata into the veg, then leave the mixture to cool completely. You can do this in advance if you like.

4 Once the filling is cool, preheat the oven to 190°C fan and line a large baking tray with baking paper. Divide the filling into 12 equal portions. Cut the sheets of pastry in half lengthways so you have two long strips. Fill the corner of one strip with a portion of filling and flip the corner inwards so all the filling is enclosed. Keep flipping the triangle over, rolling it up to completely seal in the filling in a triangle. Place on the prepared tray then, once they are all rolled, brush with the melted butter. Bake for about 25 minutes, or until the pastry is crisp and golden all over.

5 Allow to cool and store in the fridge. Enjoy cold or reheat in the microwave, or better still in the oven to crisp up the pastry again.

137
CALS

SPICY MOROCCAN CARROT DIP

PER SERVING | 137 CALS | 1G PROTEIN | 11G FAT | 7G CARBS

15 MINS   25 MINS   FREEZE

SERVES 4

250g carrots, peeled
¼ onion
2 garlic cloves, unpeeled
2½ tbsp olive oil
½ tsp ground cumin
½ tsp ground cinnamon
½ tsp salt, plus extra to taste
juice and zest of ½ orange
15g roasted hazelnuts
    or walnuts, chopped
1 tbsp harissa
½ tbsp maple syrup
1 tbsp chopped fresh
    parsley
salt, to taste

To garnish (optional)
a drizzle of olive oil
chopped fresh parsley
chopped hazelnuts

*If you don't have access
to a food processor or
blender, this dip can be
made into a salad. Once
the carrots are cooked,
toss them with the orange
zest (leave out the orange
juice), parsley, chopped
hazelnuts, olive oil, maple
syrup and salt to taste.
Garnish with parsley
and chopped hazelnuts.*

*A delicious mildly spiced dip. A perfect excuse to use up
any leftover carrots that might otherwise be thrown away.*

1 Preheat the oven to 190°C fan.

2 Chop the carrots into roughly 2cm chunks and put them in a
bowl. Add the ¼ onion (in one wedge) and the unpeeled garlic
cloves. Drizzle over 2 tbsp of the olive oil and sprinkle over the
cumin, cinnamon and salt. Mix to coat everything in the spiced
oil, then tip onto a baking tray. Roast for about 25 minutes,
stirring halfway through cooking, or until everything is tender
and beginning to caramelize. Allow to cool.

3 Once cooled, tip the carrots and onion into a food
processor. Remove the garlic cloves from their skins and
chuck those in too. Add the orange juice and zest, hazelnuts,
harissa, maple syrup and the remaining ½ tbsp of olive oil
and pulse until combined, scraping down the sides of the food
processor to make sure everything is incorporated. Once it is
homogenous, blitz in the parsley, then taste and adjust the salt
and seasonings to your liking; add more harissa if you prefer
a spicier flavour, more cinnamon for more warming flavours,
or more cumin if the depth of flavour is lacking.

4 Plate and garnish with a drizzle of olive oil and chopped
parsley and hazelnuts, if you like. Serve with crusty bread
or chopped salad veggies.

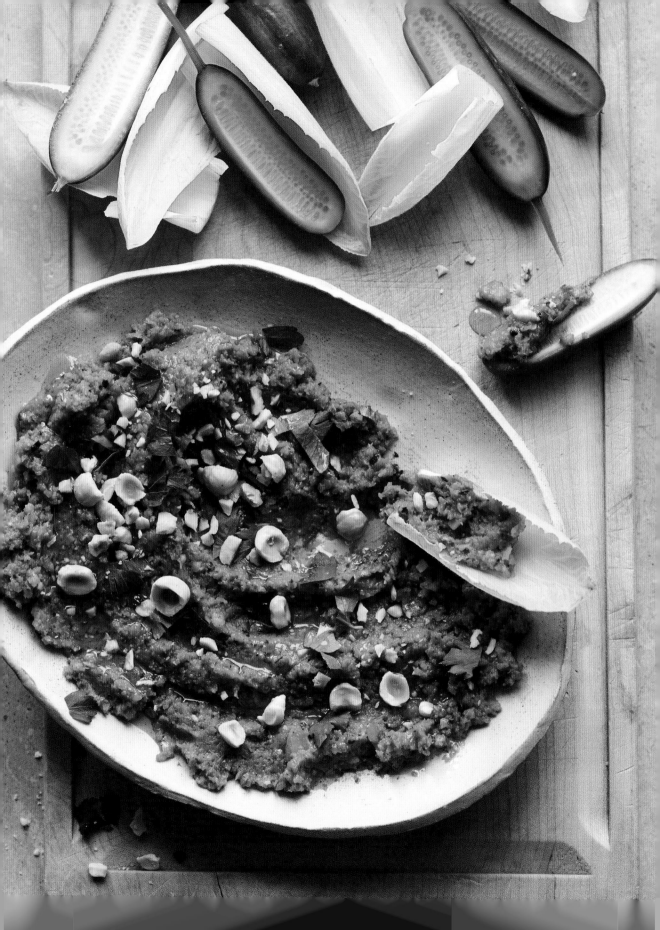

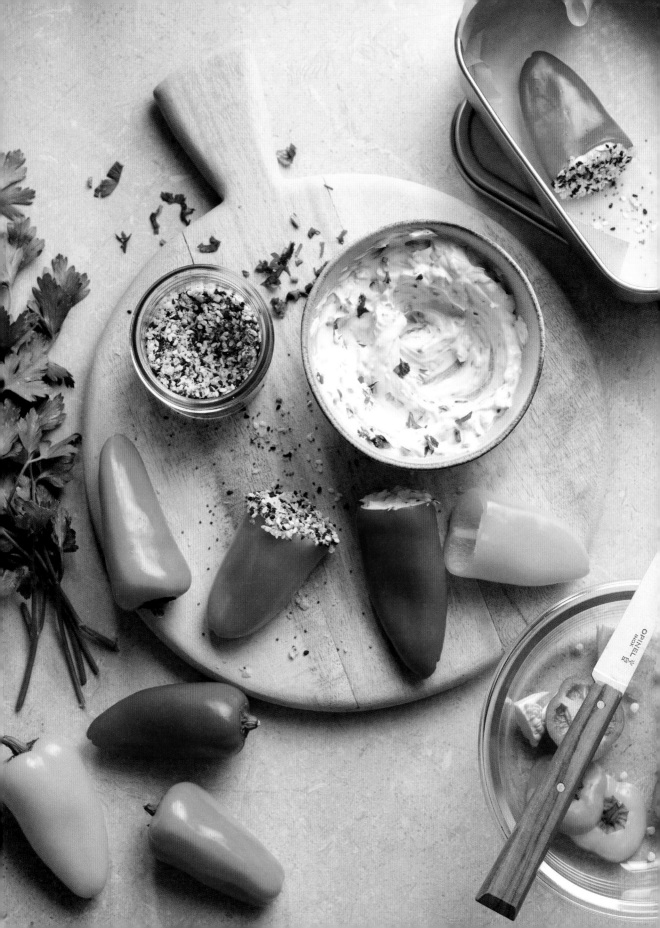

CHEESE-STUFFED MINI PEPPERS

PER SERVING | **9G** PROTEIN | **9G** FAT | **10G** CARBS

164 CALS | **prep** 15 MINS

Everything but the bagel is a seasoning mix usually found on high-calorie bagels. This does it all. Use this seasoning to get the crunch without the calories.

SERVES 2

8 mini peppers
80g low-fat cream cheese
10g fresh parsley, finely chopped

For the 'everything but the bagel' seasoning:
1 tbsp nigella (black onion) seeds
1 tbsp white sesame seeds
2 tsp poppy seeds
2 tsp garlic granules
1 tsp flaky sea salt

1 Start by making the bagel seasoning. Combine all the ingredients in a small container.

2 Use a small sharp knife to remove the stalk and hollow out each pepper, removing all the seeds.

3 Combine the cream cheese, 1½ tbsp of the seasoning and the chopped parsley and mix well.

4 Fill each mini pepper to the top with the cream cheese mixture. Press the end of each pepper into the remaining bagel seasoning so that any visible cheese is coated with the seeds.

5 Store in the fridge until ready to serve.

BAKED PARMESAN ASPARAGUS

PER SERVING | **6G** PROTEIN | **9G** FAT | **8G** CARBS

140 CALS | **prep** 10 MINS | **cook** 12 MINS

We sometimes add crispy bacon bits to this, cooking rashers until crisp, then chopping up and sprinkling over at the end. But don't forget to count the calories.

SERVES 4

400g asparagus spears
1 tbsp olive oil
20g butter, melted
2 garlic cloves, minced
30g panko breadcrumbs
a sprinkle of finely chopped fresh parsley
20g Parmesan cheese, finely grated
salt and pepper

1 Preheat the oven to 190°C fan and line a large baking tray with baking paper.

2 Chop the stalky base off the asparagus spears and place them in a large bowl. Add the oil, melted butter, garlic, breadcrumbs, parsley and cheese and season with salt and pepper. Coat the asparagus well using your hands.

3 Transfer the asparagus to the prepared tray, spreading it out in a single layer, then sprinkle any remaining mixture from the bowl across the top of the asparagus.

4 Bake for 8–10 minutes until the asparagus is tender. Finish by turning the oven to the grill setting and grilling for a couple of minutes until the asparagus and breadcrumbs are golden brown and delicious.

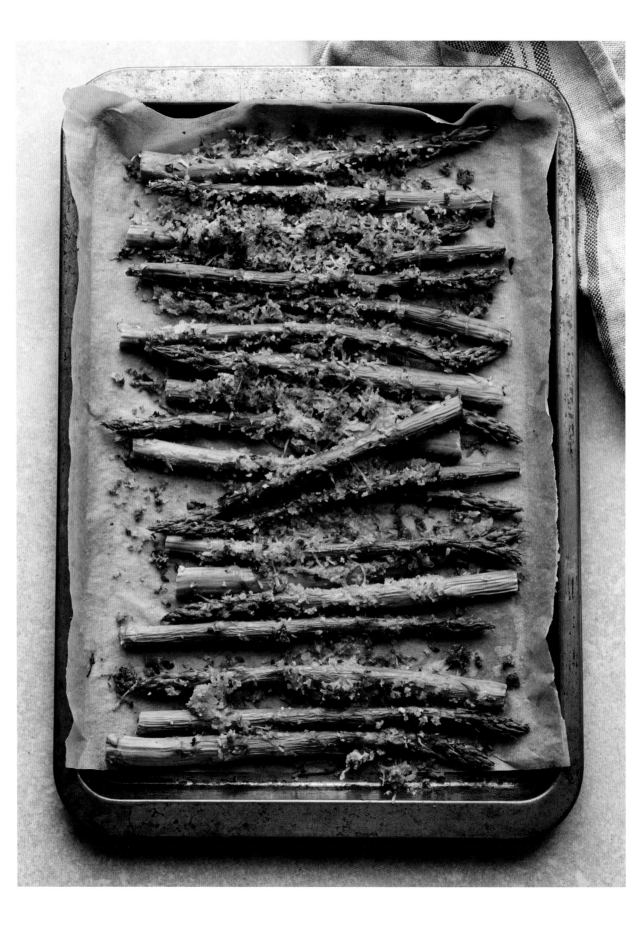

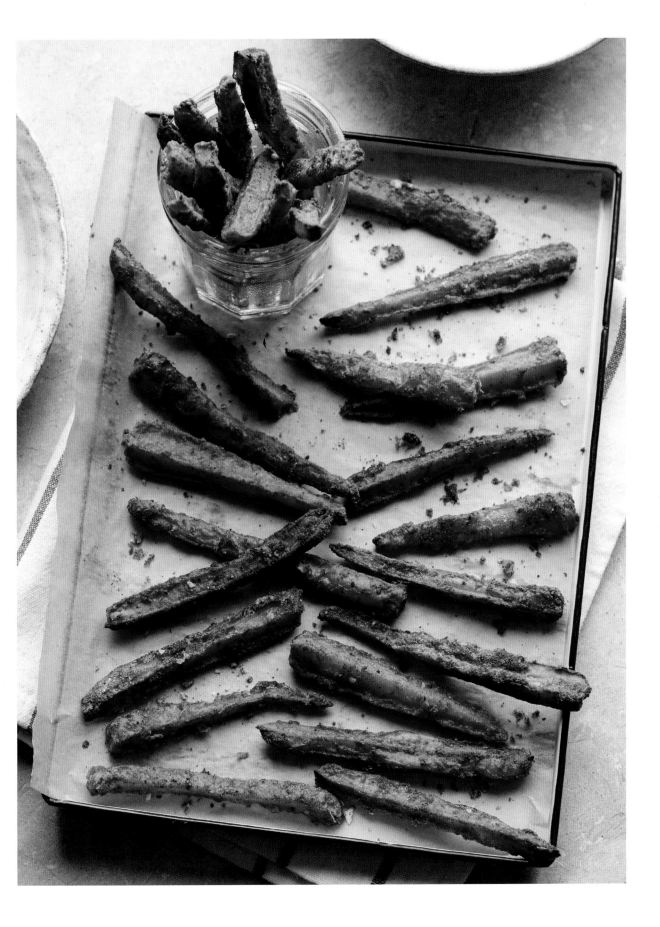

CARROT FRIES

PER SERVING | 2G PROTEIN | 13G FAT | 50G CARBS

 365 CALS **prep** 5 MINS **cook** 1 HOUR

These can't be rushed. Lower and longer seems to work best for crisp fries. You need to be patient, but they are well worth the wait.

SERVES 2

1kg large carrots, unpeeled and washed
2 tbsp olive oil
2 tbsp cornflour
¼ tsp pepper
¼ tsp salt
¼ tsp garlic granules
2 heaped tsp smoked paprika
1 tsp chilli powder (optional)
chopped fresh parsley, to garnish

1 Preheat the oven to 170°C fan and line two baking trays with baking paper.

2 Halve the carrots widthways if long. Chop the carrots into halves lengthways then half again into quarters so you get four long batons. Add to a mixing bowl and toss in the olive oil until coated.

3 Combine your cornflour and spices, then sprinkle over the carrot fries, making sure they're evenly coated. Spread out the carrots on the prepared trays, ensuring none of them are touching. Bake for about 1 hour, mixing halfway through. Check them after an hour and leave them in the oven a little longer if they are not yet crisp.

4 Once the carrots are golden and a little crispy, sprinkle with parsley and serve or leave to cool before sealing in a meal prep container and storing in the fridge.

KALE CRISPS

PER SERVING | 2G PROTEIN | 4G FAT | 1G CARBS

 46 CALS **prep** 5 MINS **cook** 15 MINS

Celery salt, garlic granules, paprika, cumin - literally any kind of seasonings work well with these. I use whatever we have. So, feel free to use what you have.

SERVES 4

200g whole leaf curly kale
1 tbsp olive oil
½ tsp smoked paprika
½ tsp garlic granules
flaky sea salt

1 Preheat the oven to 160°C fan and line two baking trays with baking paper.

2 Wash your kale and ensure it's completely dry. (If the leaves are wet, they will just steam up and we want them crispy.) Rip the leaves off the stalks so you have large pieces, getting rid of the tough centre stalk. Place into a large bowl and toss in the olive oil.

3 Tip the kale onto the prepared trays, spreading the leaves out as much as you can so they aren't overcrowded, and place in the oven for 10 minutes.

4 Take them out, giving them a good shuffle and removing any leaves that are already crisp, then place them back in the oven for another 2-5 minutes. Keep an eye on them as we want them to crisp up but not to go to dark or they can taste bitter.

5 Once cooked, sprinkle with the above seasonings or create your own. Store in a sealed airtight container until ready to eat.

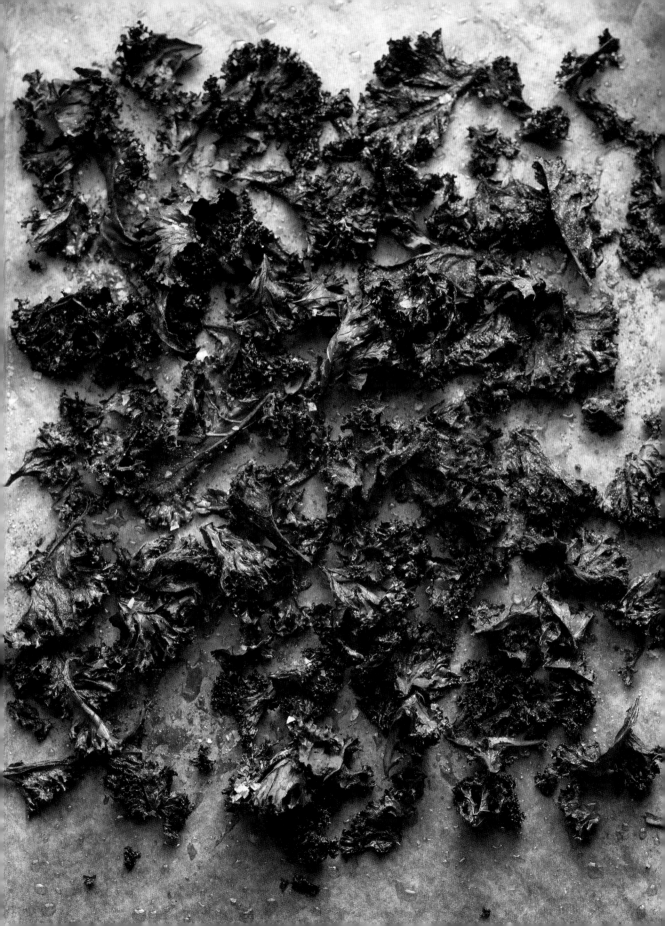

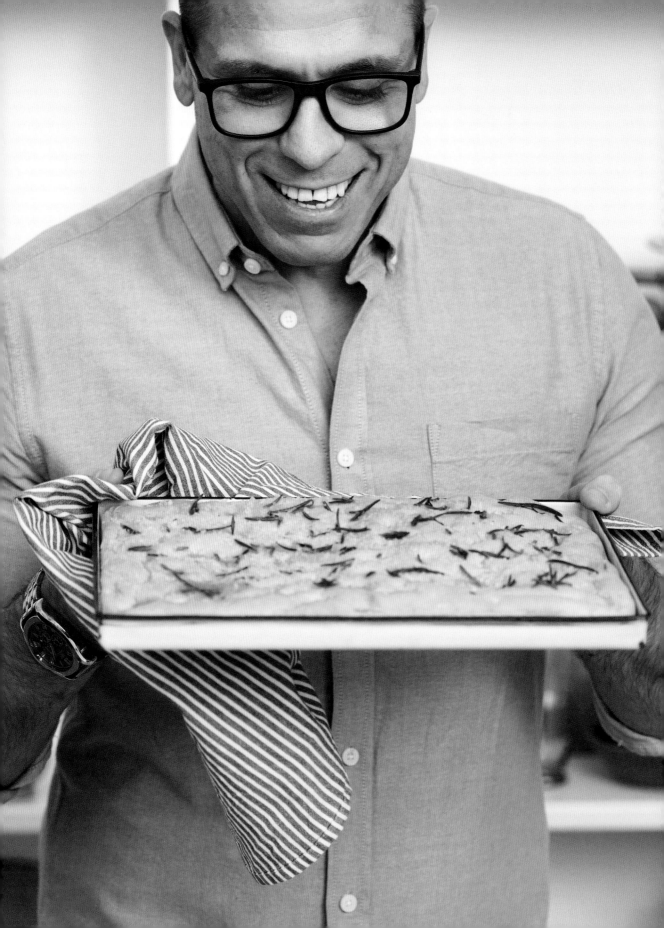

FOCACCIA GARLIC BREAD

PER SERVING | **264** CALS | **7G** PROTEIN | **8G** FAT | **41G** CARBS

prep
20 MINS +
PROVING

cook
20 MINS

FREEZE

SERVES 6

60ml olive oil, plus a drizzle
for the bowl and tray
4 garlic cloves, bashed
but still in one piece
5 sprigs fresh thyme
or 1 tbsp dried
3 sprigs fresh rosemary
or 1 tbsp dried
¼ tsp black pepper
1 x 7g sachet (or 2 tsp)
of dried yeast
¼ tsp honey
320g strong white
bread flour
½ tsp salt
1 tbsp chopped fresh
rosemary, to sprinkle
1 tsp flaked or coarse salt,
to sprinkle on top

tip

*A smaller portion will save
you some calories. Divide
it into eight pieces for
198 calories, 5g protein,
6g fat, 30g carbs.*

Did someone say garlic bread?

1 Combine the olive oil, garlic, thyme, rosemary and black
pepper in a small saucepan on low heat. Cook gently for a
couple of minutes, then turn off the heat and set aside for
the oil to infuse. You can do this in advance and give it more
time to get strongly flavoured, if you like. Once ready, remove
the garlic cloves and the herb sprigs, if using fresh.

2 In a large bowl, combine 230ml of tepid water, the yeast
and the honey. Stir a few times until the honey is dissolved,
then add about half of the flour and 1½ tbsp of the infused
olive oil. Mix together and let it sit for 8–10 minutes.

3 Stir in the remaining flour and the salt until combined.
Transfer the dough to a floured surface and knead for a few
minutes until smooth and stretchy. Or you can knead it in
a stand mixer with a dough hook attachment, if you prefer.

4 Transfer the dough to a large oiled mixing bowl, turning
the dough over to coat it with oil. Cover the bowl with a damp
towel and let it rise for 1 hour in a warm place.

5 Once the dough has finished its first rise, preheat the oven
to 230°C fan and drizzle a 22 x 32cm lipped baking tray with
a little olive oil.

6 Place the dough on the baking tray and press it down
and stretch it out to almost fill the tray. Drizzle the top of the
dough with the remaining infused oil, then use your fingers to
make dimples all over the dough. Sprinkle over the chopped
rosemary and coarse salt. Let the dough rise for another
20–25 minutes until it puffs up slightly.

7 Bake for 15–20 minutes until golden brown. Enjoy warm
or allow to cool on a wire rack. Slice into six squares.

55
CALS

BAKED-NOT-FRIED ONION BHAJIS

PER BHAJI | **55** CALS | **4G** PROTEIN | **1G** FAT | **7G** CARBS

20 MINS +
SITTING

40 MINS

FREEZE

MAKES 12

400g onions
1 tsp salt
½ tsp cumin seeds
½ tsp ground turmeric
½ tsp ground coriander
½ tsp chilli powder
a small bunch of
    fresh coriander,
    finely chopped
1 green chilli,
    finely chopped
1.5cm piece of fresh
    ginger, peeled and
    cut into very thin strips
    or coarsely grated
75g gram flour
1 tbsp vegetable oil

For the mint raita:
4 tbsp low-fat Greek yogurt
a small handful of fresh
    mint leaves, shredded
a squeeze of lemon juice
salt and pepper

tip

*You can use all white
onions for these, or
a mixture of red and
white, if you like.*

*Baking these delicious onion bhajis instead of frying them
keeps the calories low whilst keeping the amazing flavour.
Low in calories, so why not have a few?*

1 Firstly, peel and slice the onions into 3mm strips. Put the
onions in a large bowl, sprinkle with the salt and mix. Allow
to sit for at least 30 minutes. Meanwhile, preheat the oven
to 180°C fan and line a baking tray with baking paper.

2 Squeeze out the onions over the bowl to release the water,
then set aside in another bowl. Add the dried spices, fresh
coriander, chilli and ginger to the bowl with the onion water
and give the mixture a really good mix.

3 Add the onions back into the bowl and mix. Sprinkle the
gram flour over the onion mixture and mix again. There should
be enough water released from the salted onions to form a
batter that sticks the onions together. If too dry, add a drop
of water.

4 Stir the oil into the onion mixture, making sure you mix
this up so everything is covered.

5 Spoon the mixture onto the prepared baking tray to form
12 equal-sized heaps. Bake the bhajis for 35–40 minutes,
or until nicely golden.

6 While the bhajis cook, make the mint raita by combining
everything in a small bowl. Season with salt and pepper.

7 Serve the bhajis with the mint raita, or let cool and pack
into meal prep containers, with the raita stored separately.

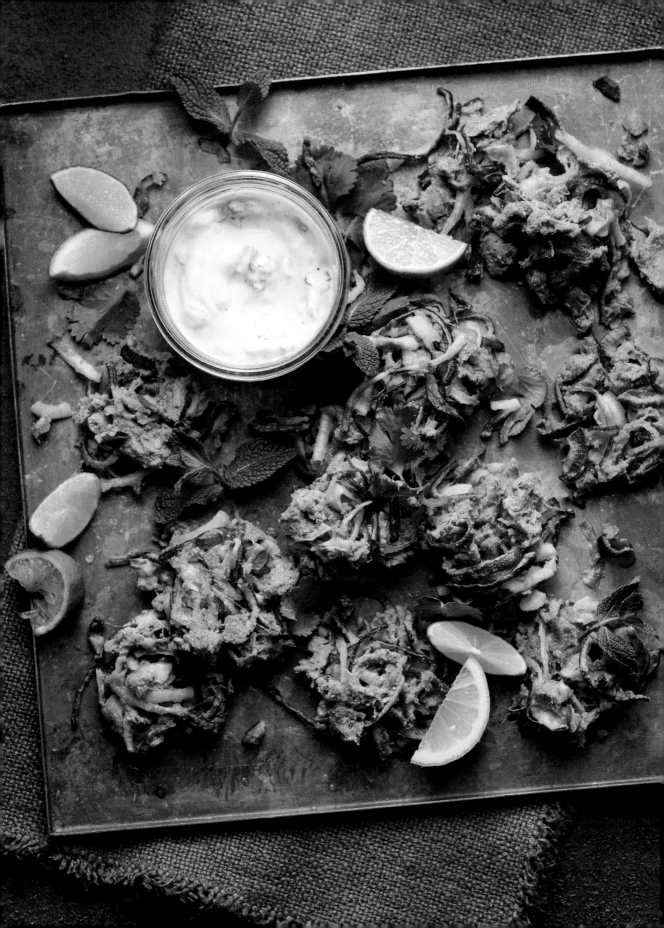

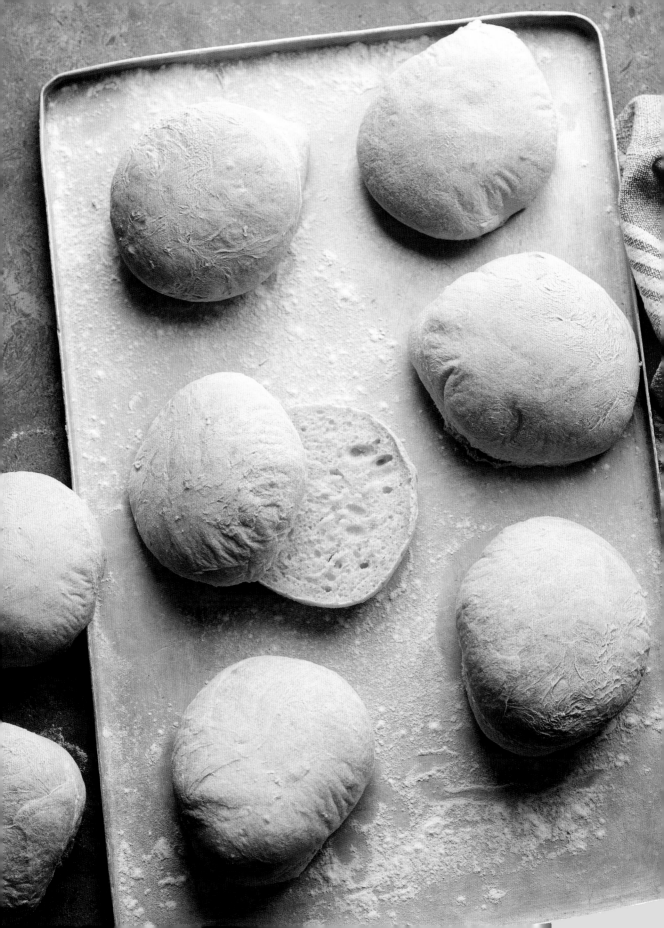

FRANK'S HOMEMADE BREAD ROLLS

PER ROLL | **211** CALS | **7G** PROTEIN | **1G** FAT | **43G** CARBS

25 MINS + **20 MINS** **FREEZE**
PROVING

MAKES 8 ROLLS

1 x 7g sachet (or 2 tsp)
  of dried yeast
½ tsp sugar
50ml skimmed milk,
  lukewarm
450g strong white bread
  flour, plus a little extra
  for dusting
1 tsp salt
a drizzle of olive oil,
  for greasing

*You can also bake the
dough in a loaf tin for
one single loaf rather
than rolls. You will need
to give it a longer cooking
time of 30-35 minutes.*

*We call these barm cakes where I'm from, but they are
basically fluffy bread rolls. They can be made by hand
if you don't have a stand mixer.*

1 Start by adding the yeast and sugar to the 50ml of tepid
milk in a small bowl. Mix until it has all dissolved, then let
sit whilst you do the next step.

2 Sift the flour into the bowl of a stand mixer fitted with a dough
hook or a large mixing bowl and stir in the salt. Make a well in
the middle of the flour and add the yeast mixture and 300ml
of tepid water. Start the mixer and allow to mix for 6-7 minutes
on the lowest setting, adding up to 100ml more water if it needs
it, until the mixture forms a smooth dough. Alternatively, bring
the mixture together with a spoon, then tip out onto a work
surface and knead by hand for 10 minutes, or until smooth
and elastic. Again, add a little more water if needs be.

3 Grease a clean mixing bowl with a little oil. Form the dough
into a ball and pop it in the greased bowl, covering the top
with cling film. Leave to prove in a warm place for 45 minutes,
or until doubled in size.

4 Once the dough has doubled in size, knead again for
4-5 minutes, knocking the air out of it. Re-cover and allow to
double in size yet again. Meanwhile, flour a large baking tray.

5 Knead the mixture one last time, then cut the dough into eight
even portions. Roll each into a smooth ball and place on the
floured tray, leaving enough space between each for them to
expand and rise. Leave to prove, covered with a tea towel, for
a final 30 minutes. Meanwhile, preheat the oven to 200°C fan.

6 Bake the rolls for 19-20 minutes, or until golden and risen.

148
CALS

SUPER GREEN SALAD

PER SERVING | **148** CALS | **8G** PROTEIN | **10G** FAT | **6G** CARBS

prep
15 MINS

cook
5 MINS

SERVES 4

300g large asparagus
    spears
90g shelled edamame
    beans
90g frozen garden peas
10g Parmesan shavings,
    to serve (optional)

For the dressing:
2¹/₂ tbsp olive oil
1 small garlic clove,
    roughly chopped
¹/₂ tsp lemon zest
1¹/₂ tbsp fresh lemon juice
a large handful of fresh
    basil leaves
a small handful of
    fresh mint leaves
salt and pepper

A bright and vibrant dish that pairs with almost anything.

1 Bring a large pan of salted water to the boil. Trim the tough ends from the asparagus. Cut half of them into 5cm lengths on the diagonal.

2 Using a vegetable peeler, shave the remaining asparagus spears into long ribbons and set aside.

3 Add the short asparagus pieces to the boiling water, along with the edamame and peas and cook for 3–4 minutes. As soon as they are tender but still have a little crunch, drain the vegetables and run under cold water to stop the cooking process. Drain and pat dry.

4 To make the dressing, put the oil, garlic and lemon zest and juice in a blender and blitz until smooth. Add the herbs and process briefly until chopped into the dressing. Season well with salt and pepper. You can also do this in a pestle and mortar.

5 Put the shaved asparagus and cooked vegetables into a serving bowl. Drizzle with the dressing and toss to coat. Top with Parmesan shavings, if you wish. If you are meal prepping this, divide it between meal prep containers and keep the dressing and Parmesan shavings in separate little containers until ready to serve.

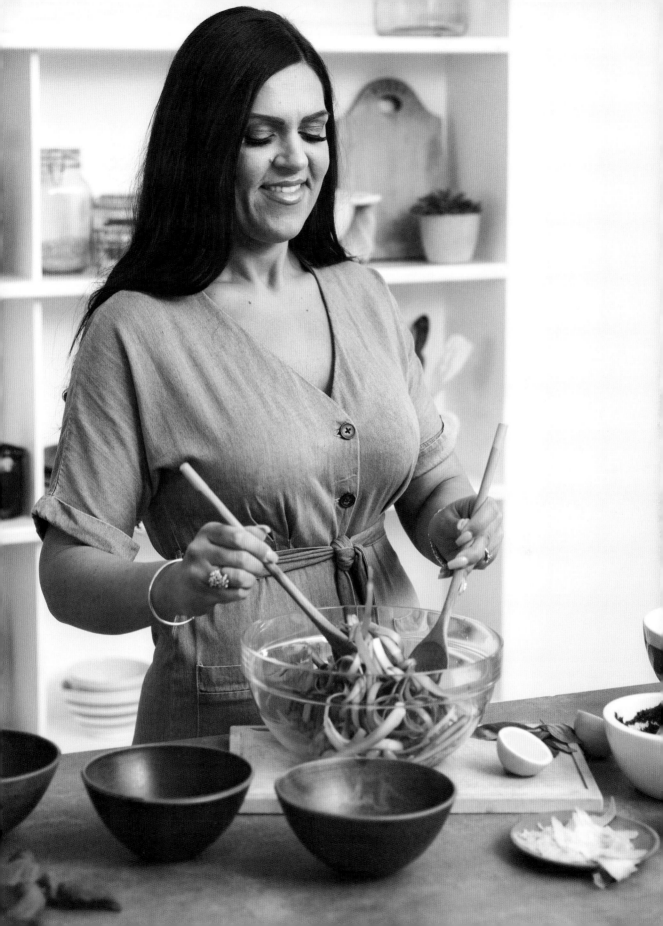

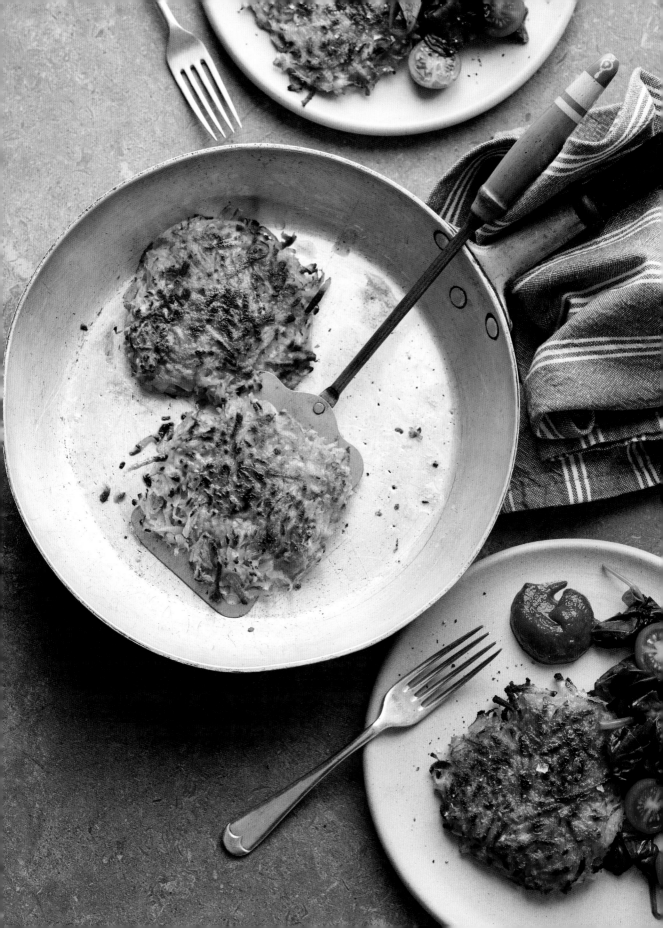

EASY HASH BROWNS

PER SERVING | 3G PROTEIN | 6G FAT | 27G CARBS

 182 CALS *prep* 20 MINS *cook* 16 MINS

These are a must as a tasty afternoon snack or side, or try with an egg for brekkie!

SERVES 4

500g potatoes, grated
2 shallots, grated
1 tbsp plain flour
a pinch of smoked paprika
¼ tsp salt
1 tbsp butter, melted
1 tbsp vegetable oil

1 Put the potatoes in a mixing bowl and cover in ice cold water to remove the starch. Give it a very good mix, then drain. Tip the potatoes onto a clean tea towel and add the shallots. Gather up the edges of the cloth, then squeeze tightly to remove as much water as you can. The more water you can get out at this step the better; squeeze and squeeze again.

2 Add the shallot and potato mixture to a mixing bowl, add the flour, paprika and salt and mix well to combine.

3 Melt half the butter with half the oil in a large non-stick frying pan on medium–high heat. Using half of the potato mixture, add two equal piles of the potato mixture to the pan and flatten down with a spatula to make patties. Fry for 3-4 minutes on each side until golden brown, pushing down with a spatula so each side is browned all over and the potato sticks together. Once cooked, transfer to a plate lined with kitchen roll and repeat to cook two more hash browns with the remaining mixture.

ROOT MASH

PER SERVING | 2G PROTEIN | 8G FAT | 16G CARBS

 160 CALS *prep* 10 MINS *cook* 20 MINS

Charlotte and I have been having this a lot lately instead of potatoes as we got a load of root veg from the market. I'll use anything: turnip, butternut squash, sweet potatoes, parsnips – the variety of concoctions is endless. We often add whatever herbs we have lying around too.

SERVES 4

500g swede
500g carrots
40g low-fat margarine
40g low-fat crème fraîche
finely chopped fresh chives or parsley
salt and pepper

1 Peel and chop your swede and carrots and add to a large pan of salted boiling water. Cook for long enough that they can be mashed – about 20 minutes – but be careful not to overcook the veg as this will make the mash a little soggy.

2 Drain off the water and leave them to steam dry in the colander for a minute or so, then tip back into the pan and add the margarine, crème fraîche and chives, and season generously. Use a potato masher to mash the veg to a chunky mash, but remember it will never be quite as smooth as potato mash!

3 Serve or divide between four meal prep containers to accompany whatever you like.

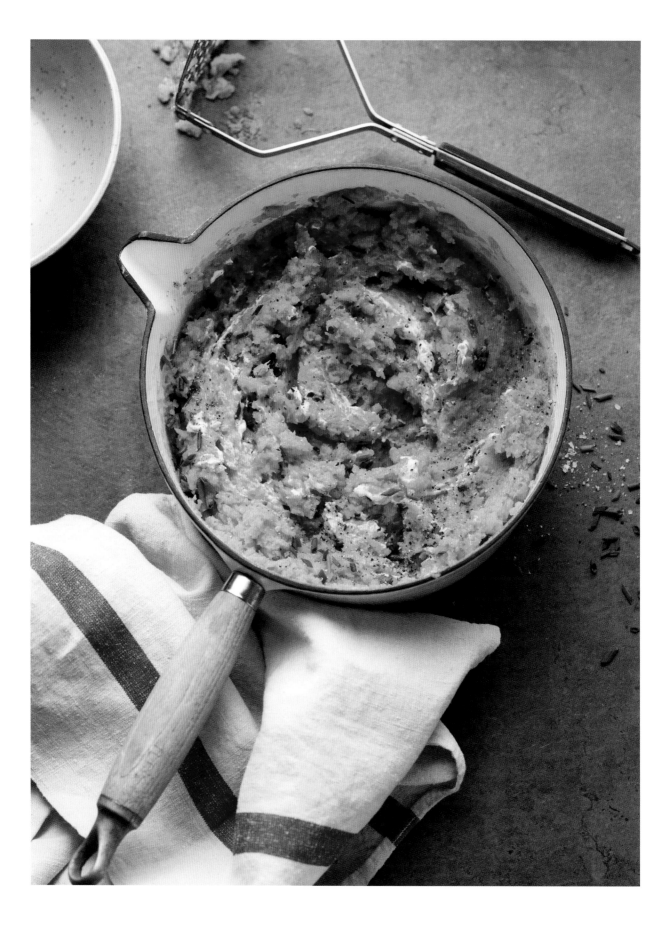

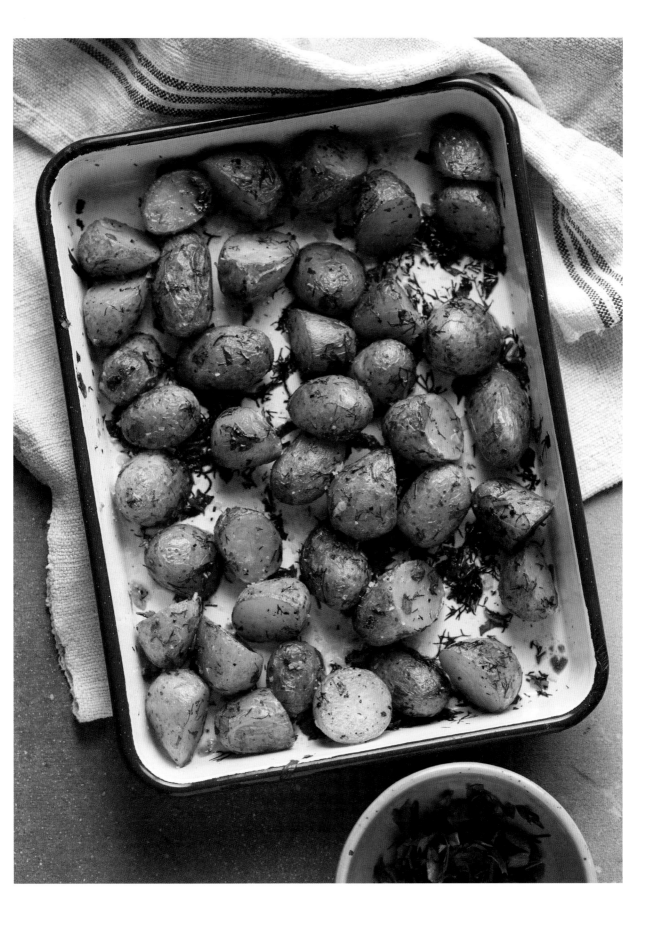

ROASTED GARLIC AND HERB POTATOES

PER SERVING | **5G** PROTEIN | **12G** FAT | **39G** CARBS

 293 CALS prep 10 MINS cook 40 MINS

Try not to eat the whole lot in one go!

SERVES 2

500g Charlotte potatoes (or scrapers)
1 tbsp olive oil
2 tsp flaked salt or ground rock salt
½ tsp pepper
2 garlic cloves, minced
1 tbsp butter, softened
a small bunch of fresh curly or
    flatleaf parsley, finely chopped
a small bunch of fresh dill, finely chopped

1 Preheat the oven to 190°C fan.

2 Wash the potatoes and slice them in half. Put them in a bowl and coat in the olive oil, salt and pepper.

3 Tip the potatoes onto a baking tray and spread out so that they are not touching one another. Roast for 30–40 minutes until golden brown and cooked through. Five minutes before the end of the cooking time, add the crushed garlic to the tray and mix around to coat the potatoes, then return the tray for the remaining time to the oven to cook the garlic a little.

4 Once cooked, transfer the potatoes to a bowl and add the butter, parsley and dill. Toss to melt the butter and coat the potatoes, then season to your liking. If you are meal prepping, store the herbs and butter separately and stir them in just before eating, once you have reheated the potatoes.

NAAN BREADS

PER BREAD | **9G** PROTEIN | **4G** FAT | **40G** CARBS

 234 CALS prep 10 MINS cook 25 MINS

A great alternative to store-bought naan breads, with only five ingredients.

MAKES 4

200g self-raising flour, plus extra for dusting
170g fat-free Greek yogurt
1 tbsp salted butter
2 tsp finely chopped fresh coriander
flaky sea salt

1 Combine the flour, yogurt and a good pinch of salt in a large mixing bowl using a wooden spoon. Add a little water if you need to bring the dough together, but don't make it too sticky – it still needs to be firm enough to roll out. Turn out onto a lightly floured surface and knead for 3–5 minutes until you have a nice, smooth dough.

2 Divide the dough into four equal portions. Using a rolling pin, roll out the dough to a flatbread about 15–18cm long. It doesn't really matter what shape it is, as long as it will fit in your pan.

3 Heat a large non-stick frying pan on medium heat. Add a piece of dough and cook for 2–3 minutes on each side until bubbling up. You want to see some definite dark brown spots before you flip. Repeat to cook all the breads.

4 Melt the butter, then stir in the chopped coriander. Brush each naan bread with the butter, then sprinkle with salt and enjoy.

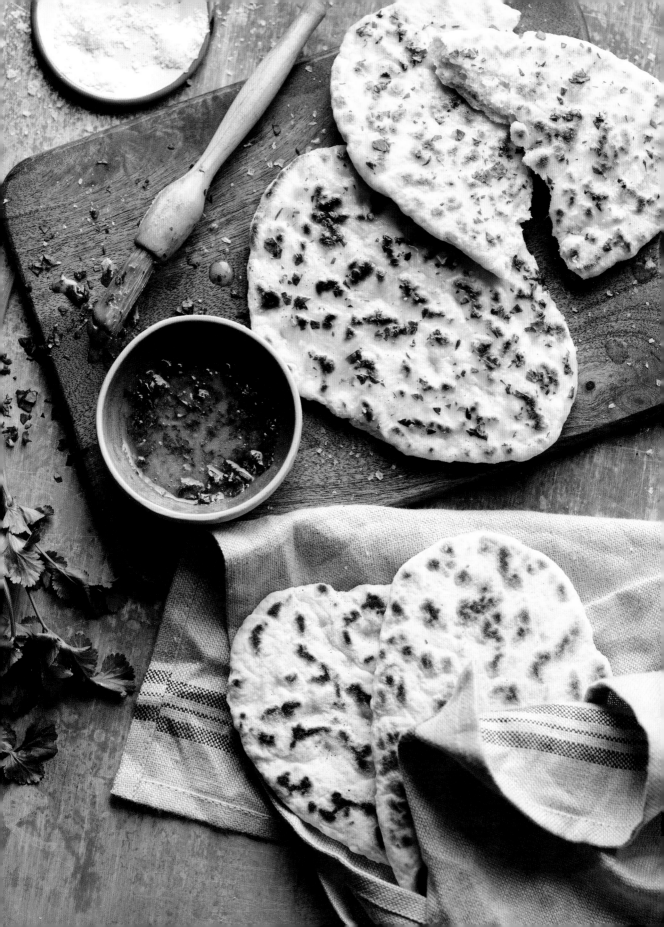

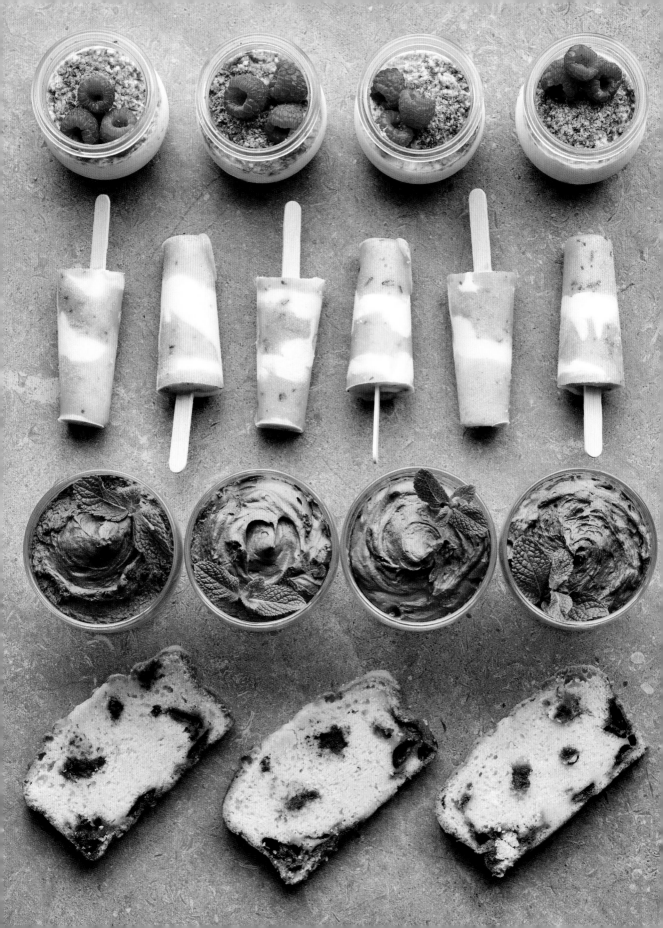

SWEET THINGS

67
CALS

MELON AND GRAPEFRUIT SALAD

PER SERVING | **67** CALS | **1G** PROTEIN | **0G** FAT | **14G** CARBS

prep

10 MINS

SERVES 4

1 medium-sized melon
    (such as galia, honeydew,
    cantaloupe)
2 pink grapefruit
8 tbsp unsweetened
    fresh orange juice
a drizzle of honey
fresh mint leaves,
    to garnish

There's something to be said for eating colourful food. This dish is packed with healthy ingredients that will leave you feeling refreshed.

1 Cut the melon into segments and deseed. Dice up the fruit, removing the skin as you go, and place into meal prep containers or a serving bowl.

2 Slice off the top and bottom of each grapefruit so it sits flat, then run a small, sharp knife down the sides to remove the skin. Cut out the segments of flesh on either side of each membrane, leaving the membrane behind. Add the segments and any juice to the melon.

3 Pour in the orange juice and finish with a drizzle of honey and a garnish of fresh mint. Best served cold from the fridge.

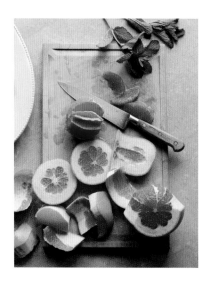

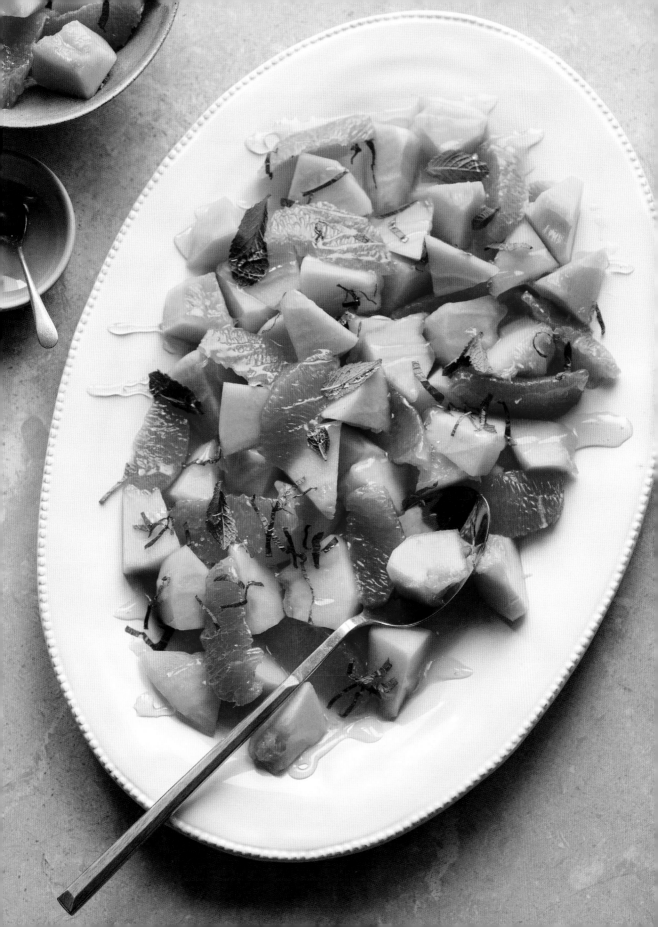

210

CALS

HONEY AND RAISIN BISCUITS

PER BISCUIT | **210** CALS | **6G** PROTEIN | **9G** FAT | **26G** CARBS

prep
20 MINS

cook
13 MINS

FREEZE

MAKES 12

30g coconut oil
60g butter
120g honey
240g porridge oats
50g whey protein
   (strawberry chocolate
   or vanilla flavour)
1 tsp ground cinnamon
100g raisins

Who doesn't love a good biscuit? A super-quick and easy recipe that the whole family can enjoy.

1 Preheat the oven to 180°C fan and line a baking sheet with non-stick baking paper.

2 Melt the coconut oil, butter and honey in a saucepan, stirring continuously.

3 Put the oats, whey protein and cinnamon in a food processor and pour in the melted butter mixture. Blend until everything is well combined.

4 Once everything is mixed, add the raisins and stir through by hand. It's important not to combine them with the food processor or the raisins will be chopped and blended in and you want them whole.

5 Tip the biscuit mixture onto the prepared baking sheet and form into a rough rectangle. Lay another sheet of baking paper over the top and roll out until about 5mm thick. Peel off the paper and tidy up the edges a little by pressing them back into a straight line with the side of a long knife. Bake for 10 minutes, then remove from the oven and let cool for a couple of minutes. Slice the rectangle to divide it into 12 biscuits, spacing them out a little by sliding them apart with the knife. Return the tray to the oven for a further 2–3 minutes, until golden all over. They will be quite crumbly when hot, so allow to cool before removing from the baking sheet.

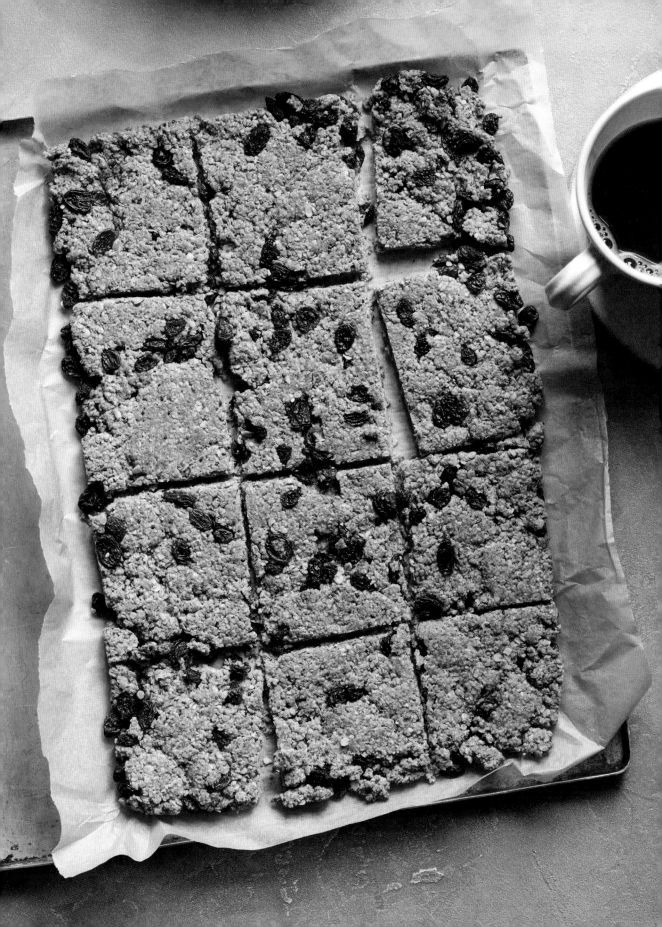

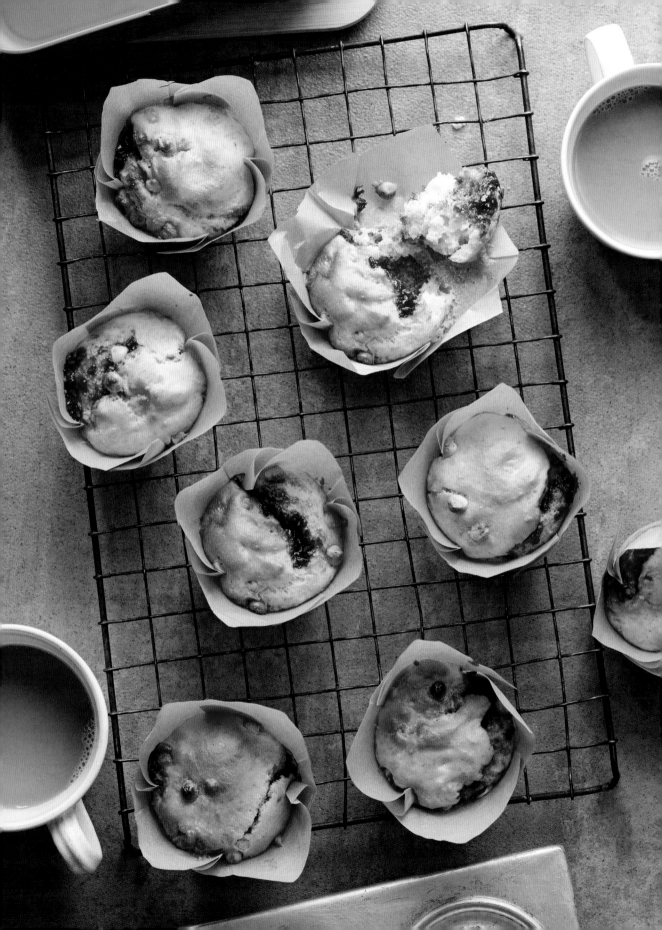

202
CALS

WHITE CHOCOLATE RASPBERRY MUFFINS

PER MUFFIN | **202** CALS | **4G** PROTEIN | **6G** FAT | **32G** CARBS

prep
15 MINS

cook
25 MINS

FREEZE

MAKES 8

200g self-raising flour
½ tsp baking powder
50g caster sugar
¼ tsp salt
1 medium egg
30ml vegetable oil
120ml skimmed milk
50g white chocolate
   chips
80g low-sugar
   raspberry jam

Who said you can't have your cake and eat it? These muffins are sure to hit the spot!

1 Preheat the oven to 170°C fan and line a muffin tray with eight non-stick paper cases.

2 Sift the flour and baking powder into a large bowl and add the sugar and salt. Stir to combine.

3 In a large jug, whisk together the egg, oil and milk, then pour this into the flour mixture. Tip in the chocolate chips, then fold the mixture gently until it's just coming together – a few lumps are fine.

4 Divide most of the batter between the cake cases, stopping when you have about a quarter of the mixture left. Using a teaspoon to spoon it in, divide the jam between the cupcake cases, then divide out the remaining batter to almost cover the jam.

5 Bake in the centre of the oven for 20–25 minutes until risen and golden.

6 Try not to eat them all at once.

182
CALS

PEANUT BUTTER CUPS

PER SERVING | **182** CALS | **3G** PROTEIN | **13G** FAT | **12G** CARBS

20 MINS +
FREEZING   5 MINS   FREEZE

MAKES 8 OR 16 MINI

130g milk or dark chocolate
2 tbsp melted coconut oil
65g peanut butter
30g honey
a pinch of rock salt, plus
    a sprinkle for the tops

If you are using little petit four cases, a serving is two cups. For the larger cupcake cases, just have the one. They are so rich they will really hit the spot!

These are perfect for those with a sweet tooth. Great to keep you on track while still getting that sweet fix!

1 Line a bun tray with eight fairy cake cases or a mini muffin tray with 16 petit four cases.

2 Melt the chocolate and 1 tbsp of the coconut oil together in the microwave. Blitz for 30 seconds at a time, stirring in between, until smooth and runny. If you don't have a microwave, put the chocolate in a glass or ceramic bowl set over a pan of hot water to melt.

3 Divide about half of the chocolate between the paper liners and chill for 10 minutes until the chocolate has set.

4 In another bowl, combine the peanut butter, remaining 1 tbsp of coconut oil, honey and rock salt and microwave, in short blasts again and stirring each time, until the mixture slightly melts and is pourable.

5 Remove the tray from the freezer then pour the peanut butter mixture into the holes, dividing it evenly between the liners. Place back into the fridge for 10 minutes.

6 Once set, pour in the remaining chocolate so it covers the peanut butter in each liner. Add a sprinkle of rock salt then place back into the freezer for 1 hour.

7 These can be stored in the fridge or freezer. Please note, at room temperature these will melt due to the coconut oil. And if storing them in the freezer, leave for about 5 minutes to soften before eating.

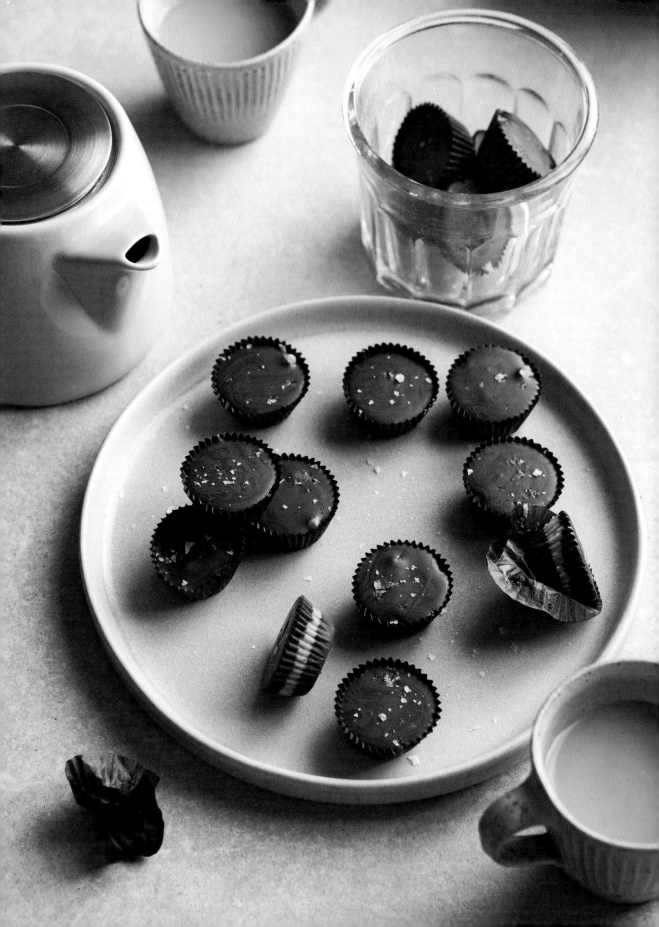

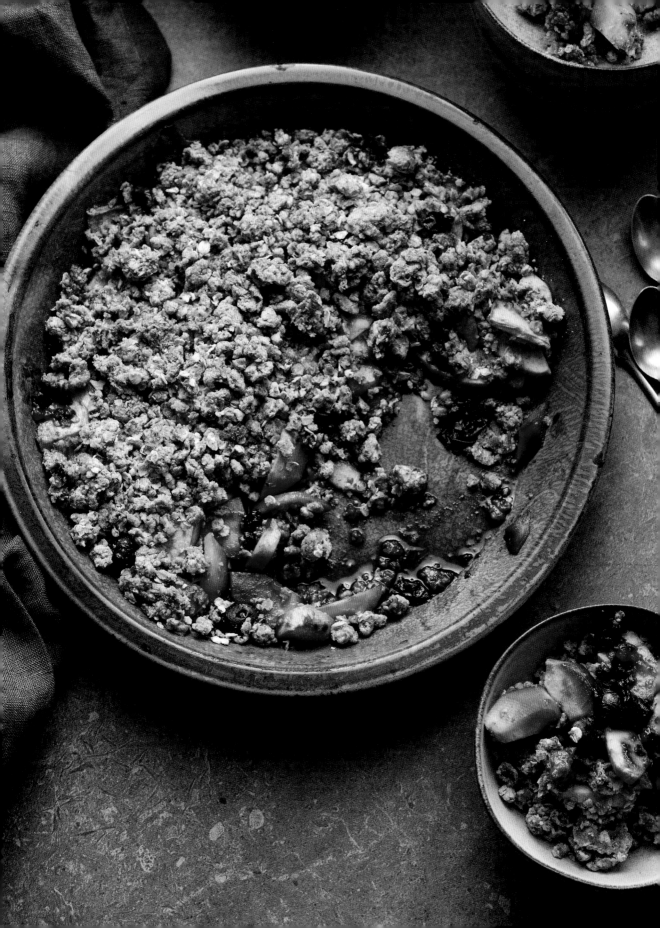

BLUEBERRY AND APPLE OATMEAL CRUMBLE

PER SERVING | 304 CALS | 6G PROTEIN | 10G FAT | 45G CARBS

15 MINS   40 MINS   FREEZE

SERVES 4

75g wholemeal flour
50g rolled oats
50g brown sugar
1 tsp ground cinnamon
25g ground almonds
50g low-fat margarine
200g blueberries (fresh
  or frozen and defrosted)
3 eating apples, peeled
  and thinly sliced
1 tsp honey
fat-free Greek yogurt,
  to serve (optional)

An old-fashioned favourite that's still as popular today! Great served with a swirl of low-fat squirty cream.

1 Preheat the oven to 180°C fan.

2 Put the flour, oats, sugar, cinnamon and almonds in a bowl and stir to combine. Rub the low-fat margarine into the mixture with your fingertips until it resembles breadcrumbs.

3 Divide the blueberries and apples into four separate ramekins, or one ovenproof dish, about 20cm x 20cm. Drizzle the honey over the fruit and stir to mix.

4 Spoon the crumble over the individual ramekins or ovenproof dish, making sure to evenly cover.

5 Bake for 40 minutes, or until the crumble is golden and the fruit is cooked and bubbling. Serve with yogurt, if you like.

51 CALS

PEACHES AND CREAM LOLLIES

PER LOLLY | **51** CALS | **2G** PROTEIN | **1G** FAT | **7G** CARBS

20 MINS +
FREEZING   **5 MINS**   **FREEZE**

MAKES 8

2 large peaches,
   destoned and sliced
juice of ½ lemon
3 tbsp maple syrup
1 tsp vanilla extract
1 tbsp powdered or
   granulated sweetener
180g Greek yogurt

At only 51 calories a lolly, these are great to have after
any meal. Why not double up on the ingredients and keep
a stash in the freezer?

1 Put the sliced peaches and lemon juice into a small saucepan
over medium heat. Cook them down until slightly softened.
You still want to preserve some of the fresh peach flavours,
so don't cook them so much that they go to a mush.

2 Once softened, blend or place in a food processor with
1 tbsp of the maple syrup. Blend until smooth, then set aside
to cool.

3 Stir the remaining maple syrup, the vanilla extract and
the sweetener into the yogurt until thoroughly combined.

4 Layer the peach purée and sweetened yogurt into ice
lolly moulds until you reach the top. Place in the freezer
and freeze until the lollies are set.

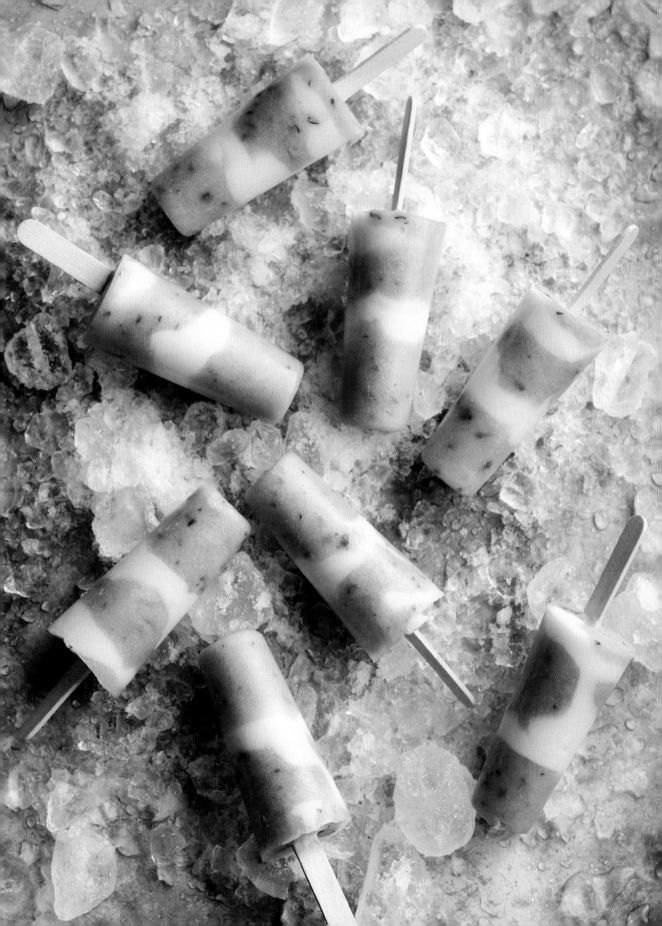

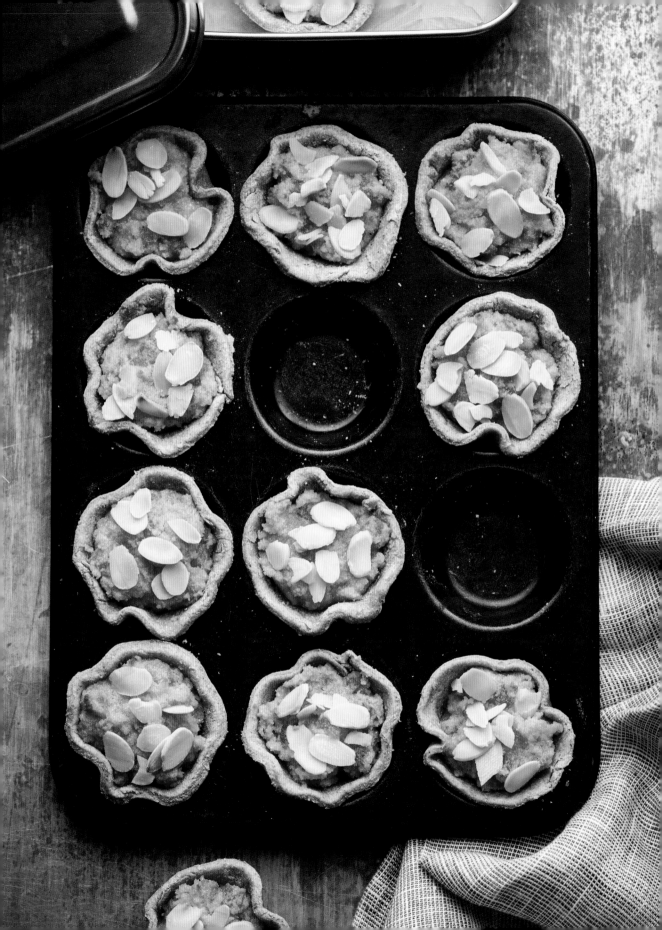

APRICOT AND ALMOND TARTS

PER TART | **178** CALS | **4G** PROTEIN | **10G** FAT | **16G** CARBS

25 MINS +
CHILLING   18 MINS   FREEZE

MAKES 12

For the pastry:
75g low-fat margarine
180g wholemeal flour

For the filling:
50g margarine
1 egg
2 tbsp honey
70g ground almonds
½ tsp almond extract
75g soft dried apricots,
 chopped
15g flaked almonds

A delicious little treat that can be eaten at any time of the day. They are also great to share – why not take some to work to share with friends and colleagues?

1 Preheat the oven to 170°C fan.

2 Add the margarine, 3 tbsp of water and about 2 tbsp of the flour to a large mixing bowl and mix with a fork. Add the rest of the flour and combine to create a stiff dough. If you need to, add a further 1 tbsp water to bring the mixture together into a ball. Wrap in cling film and chill for 30 minutes.

3 For the filling, combine the margarine, egg, honey, ground almonds and almond extract until blended, then stir in the apricots.

4 Roll out the pastry very thinly and use a 7.5cm cookie or pastry cutter to stamp out 12 circles. Use the circles to line a shallow bun tin, making sure to push them up at the sides to make a pastry casing.

5 Divide the filling between the pastry cases and sprinkle the tops with flaked almonds. Bake for 16–18 minutes, until the filling is risen and golden. Allow to cool in the tin for a few minutes before moving to a wire rack to cool completely.

299
CALS

BLUEBERRY LEMON CAKE

PER SLICE | **299** CALS | **6G** PROTEIN | **14G** FAT | **37G** CARBS

prep 20 MINS   cook 1 HOUR   FREEZE

MAKES 1 LOAF (12 SLICES)

170g unsalted butter,
   at room temperature
225g caster sugar
finely grated zest of
   2 small lemons and
   the juice of 1
4 large eggs, at room
   temperature
1½ tsp vanilla extract
250g plain flour
2 tsp baking powder
½ tsp bicarbonate of soda
½ tsp salt
110ml full-fat milk,
   at room temperature
150g fresh or frozen
   blueberries (fresh
   work best)

Blueberries and lemon: what a great combo! Just try not to eat the whole cake. Remember those calories.

1 Preheat the oven to 160°C fan.

2 Grease and line a 23 x 13cm loaf tin with baking paper, allowing the shorter sides to extend 5cm past the sides for easy removal of the loaf once baked. Set aside.

3 Put the butter, sugar and lemon zest into the bowl of a stand mixer fitted with a paddle attachment and mix together until light and fluffy, about 2 minutes.

4 Add one egg at a time, scraping down the bowl between each addition. Add the vanilla and mix until well combined.

5 Set aside 2 tbsp of the flour, then sift the rest into a medium-sized bowl and stir in the baking powder, bicarbonate of soda and salt. Add the flour mixture to the batter, alternating with the milk. Use a low speed until just a few streaks of flour are visible and be careful not to overmix.

6 Combine the blueberries with the reserved 2 tbsp of flour. Gently fold the blueberries into the batter using a spatula or wooden spoon. Do not over mix. Transfer the batter to the prepared loaf tin.

7 Bake for about 1 hour, or until the top is golden brown and a toothpick inserted into the centre comes out clean or with a few crumbs remaining. If the cake is browning too quickly on top, cover loosely with a piece of kitchen foil.

8 Remove the cake from the oven and allow to cool in the baking tin for 10 minutes. Use the baking paper ends to remove the loaf and cool completely on a wire rack.

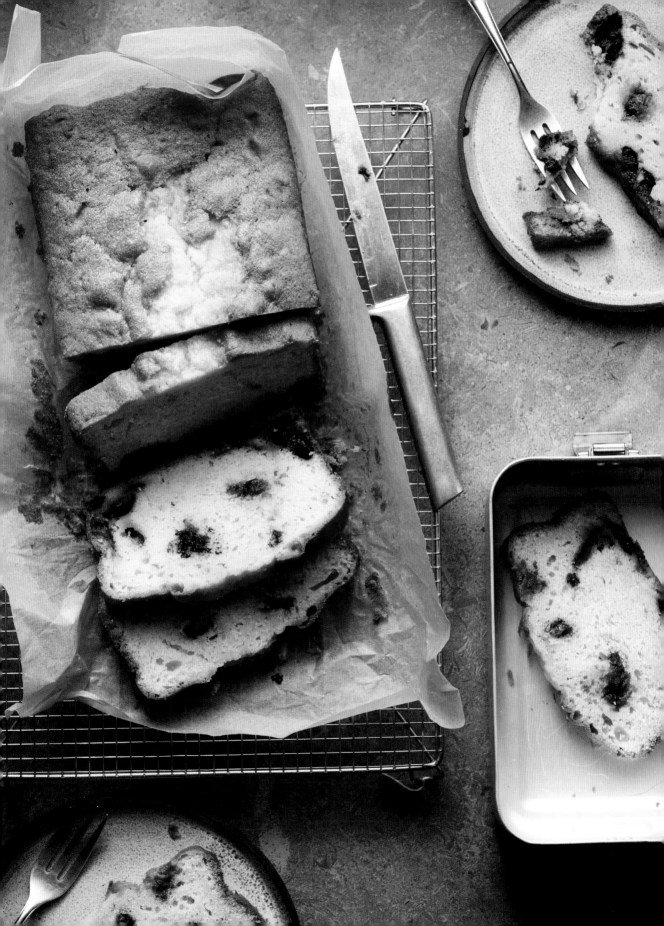

234 CALS

RICE PUDDING

PER SERVING | **234** CALS | **6G** PROTEIN | **8G** FAT | **34G** CARBS

prep
10 MINS

cook
1 HOUR
15 MINS

FREEZE

SERVES 4

100g pudding rice
30g soft brown sugar
550ml whole milk
2 tsp vanilla extract
15g butter, plus extra
    for greasing
a good pinch of
    ground nutmeg
a good pinch of
    ground cinnamon
fresh raspberries, crushed,
    to serve (optional)

I absolutely love rice pudding cold out of a tin. But there's nothing as good as homemade rice pudding. Nothing even comes close!

1 Preheat the oven 160°C fan and grease a small–medium baking dish with a little butter (or use individual ramekins).

2 Put the rice, sugar, milk and vanilla extract in the ovenproof dish and give it a stir. Add the butter, breaking it into small pieces and letting it sit on the top.

3 Put in the oven for 45 minutes then remove and break the skin. Stir, then sprinkle the top with the spices and place back into the oven for another 30 minutes.

4 The top should have a nice golden skin when finished and the rice will be tender. Serve topped with a few crushed fresh raspberries, if you like. To reheat, cover and pop in the microwave; add a splash more milk if it looks a little dry.

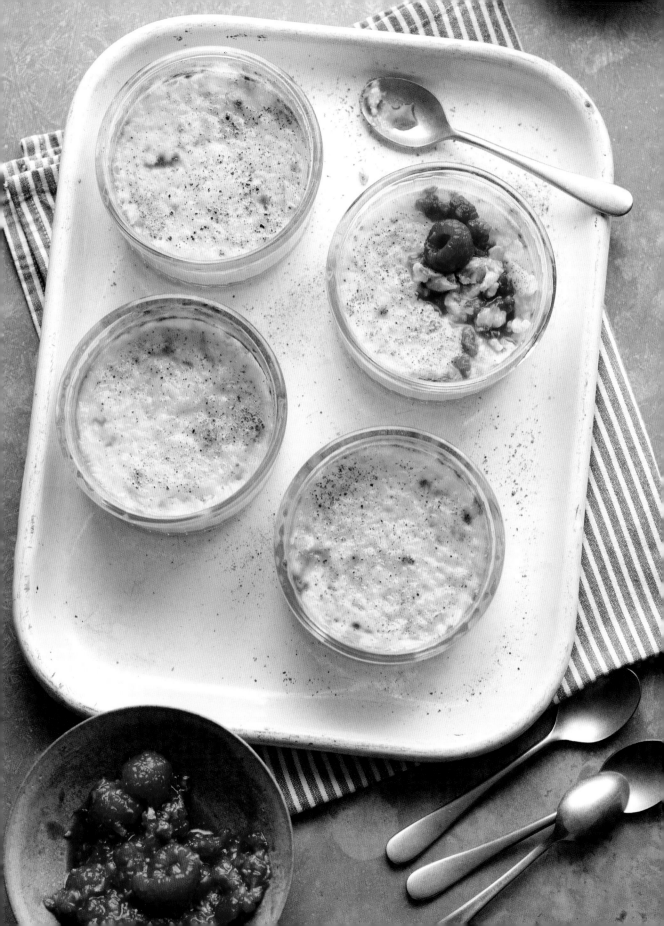

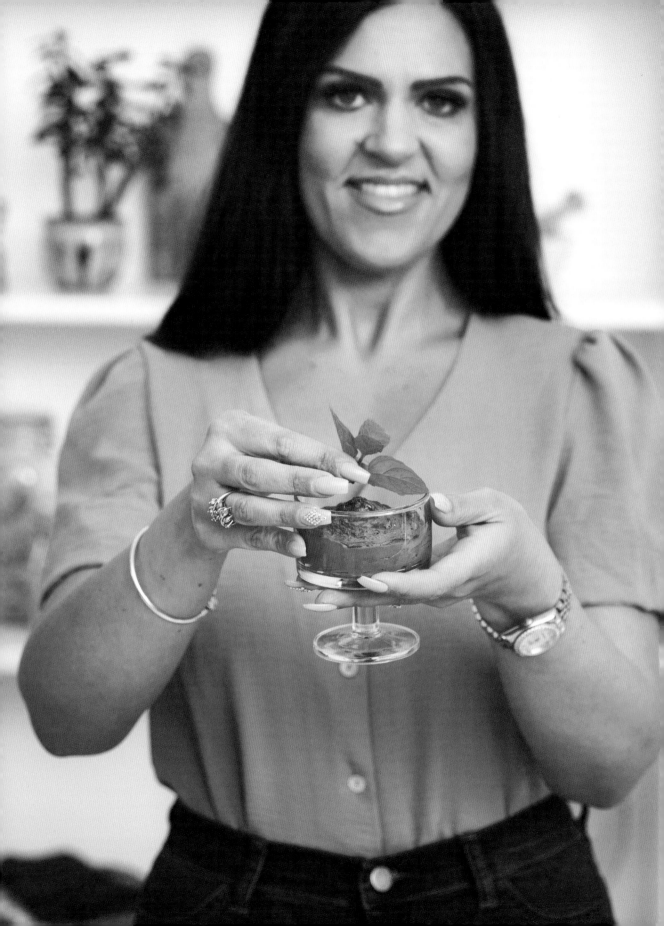

MINT CHOC MOUSSE

PER SERVING | **201** CALS | **4G** PROTEIN | **7G** FAT | **30G** CARBS

prep 10 MINS   cook 5 MINS

SERVES 4

100g very dark chocolate
   (85% cocoa solids),
   broken up
1 tsp mint extract
3 large egg whites,
   at room temperature
60g caster sugar
fresh mint sprigs, to
   decorate (optional)

*Whip up this decadent chocolate dessert in no time.
A stand mixer is useful for this, or just an extra pair of hands!*

1 Put the chocolate in a heatproof bowl with the mint extract and melt it either in short bursts in the microwave, stirring in between, or by suspending the bowl over a pan of simmering water. Once melted, remove from the heat and leave to cool a little, but so that it is still runny.

2 After the chocolate has been cooling for a few minutes, put the egg whites in a large mixing bowl and whisk with an electric hand whisk or in a stand mixer until they are frothy and beginning to form peaks. Start adding the sugar, a spoonful at a time, while whisking. Once all the sugar is added, keep whisking until you have a firm meringue. Test it's ready by rubbing a little between your finger and thumb – it shouldn't feel grainy at all.

3 With the mixer still running on high speed, start to trickle the chocolate into the meringue mixture. Once it's all added, stop whisking and scrape down the sides of the bowl with a spatula and quickly fold any unmixed chocolate in. Spoon the mousse into four bowls or meal prep containers and keep in the fridge until ready to serve. Decorate the tops with sprigs of mint, if you wish.

260
CALS

LEMON 'CHEESECAKE' JARS

PER SERVING | **260** CALS | **25G** PROTEIN | **8G** FAT | **20G** CARBS

prep

10 MINS

SERVES 4

800g fat-free Greek yogurt
finely grated zest of
2 lemons
1–2 tbsp powdered
sweetener
60g honey
1 tbsp vanilla extract
80g milled flaxseed/linseed
fresh raspberries, for
topping (optional)

tip

*If you prefer, you can top
the jars with desiccated
coconut instead of
milled flaxseed.*

*The combination of flaxseed, sweetened yogurt and berries
really does make you feel like you're eating a high calorie
cheesecake – without the excess calories of course!*

1 Put the yogurt, lemon zest, 1 tbsp of the sweetener, honey
and vanilla extract in a mixing bowl and stir well. You may
want to add more sweetener depending on your taste.

2 Divide the yogurt mixture between four bowls or jars
and top with the milled flaxseed, dividing it equally between
the portions. Scatter over a few fresh raspberries to serve,
if you like.

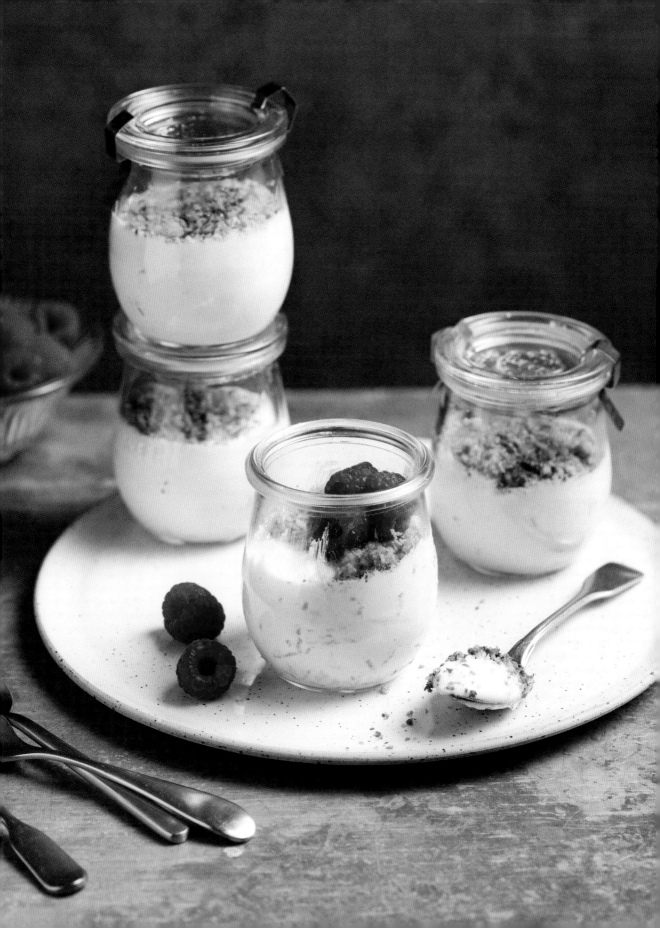

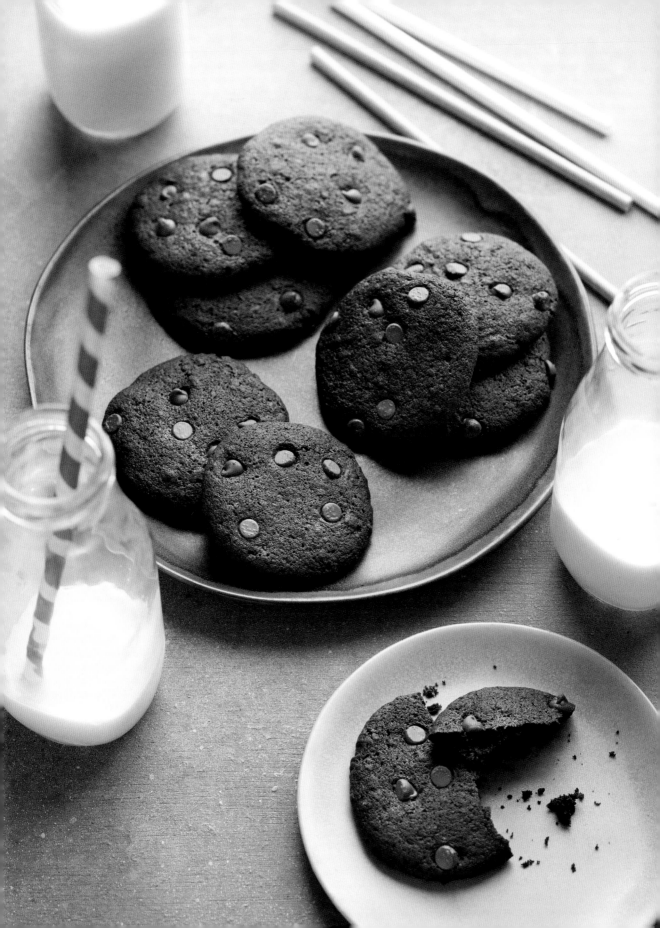

DOUBLE CHOCOLATE COOKIES

PER COOKIE | **144** CALS | **3G** PROTEIN | **8G** FAT | **14G** CARBS

10 MINS   9 MINS   FREEZE

MAKES 12

75g plain flour
30g unsweetened
  cocoa powder
¼ tsp bicarbonate
  of soda
¼ tsp salt
100g milk chocolate
  chips, plus 25g extra
  for the tops
60g unsalted butter
40g brown sugar
1 large egg
1 tsp vanilla extract

The whole family will love these. Great for a lunch box treat or eating on the go!

1 Preheat the oven to 180°C fan and line a baking tray with baking paper.

2 Start by adding the flour, cocoa powder, bicarbonate of soda and salt to a mixing bowl. Stir to combine.

3 In another large heatproof bowl, melt the milk chocolate – either in short blasts in the microwave, stirring between, or by setting the bowl above a pan of simmering water.

4 Add the butter, sugar, egg and vanilla extract to the melted chocolate and mix until everything is well combined. Now add the dry ingredients and stir everything together, taking care not to over mix.

5 Using a tablespoon or ice cream scoop, spoon the dough onto the prepared baking tray, leaving around 5cm of space between each cookie. Finally, press some extra chocolate chips on top.

6 Bake in the middle of the preheated oven for 9 minutes for fudgy cookies, or for a couple of minutes longer for crisper cookies. Remove from the oven and leave to cool on the tray for 5 minutes before transferring to a wire rack. Enjoy slightly warm or cold.

267 CALS

DATE AND OAT SLICES

PER SLICE | **267** CALS | **4G** PROTEIN | **13G** FAT | **32G** CARBS

prep 20 MINS *cook* 40 MINS FREEZE

MAKES 14

250g dried dates, chopped
3 tbsp apple juice
175ml sunflower oil
4 tbsp honey
175g wholemeal flour
175g whole rolled oats
50g walnuts, chopped

These are a lovely energy boost if you don't like your treats overly sweet.

1 Preheat the oven to 180°C fan and grease and line a 20cm square cake tin.

2 Put the dates and the apple juice in a saucepan and simmer for 6–8 minutes until the dates are soft.

3 Put the oil and honey into a separate large saucepan and stir on a low heat until blended. Add the flour, oats and walnuts to the pan and mix together thoroughly.

4 Pour half the mixture into the cake tin and press it down firmly – a potato masher is useful for this. Spoon the date mixture on top and spread out evenly. Add the remaining oat mixture and press this down firmly using whatever you have to smooth it out, such as a stepped palette knife, or the potato masher again.

5 Bake for about 30 minutes until golden brown.

6 Leave to cool in the tin for a few minutes before transferring to a wire rack to cool completely. Slice the large square in half, then slice each half into seven slices.

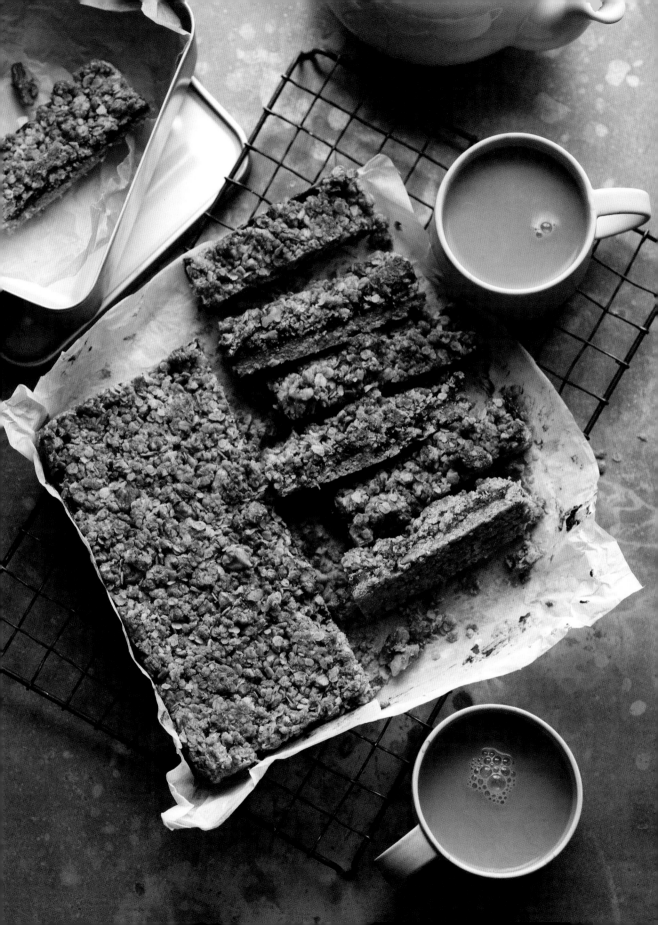

109
CALS

AVOCADO CHOCOLATE TRUFFLES

PER TRUFFLE | **109** CALS | **4G** PROTEIN | **8G** FAT | **6G** CARBS

20 MINS +   5 MINS   FREEZE
CHILLING

MAKES 12

150g avocado flesh,
    roughly chopped
40g chocolate protein
    powder
1 tsp vanilla extract
½ tsp almond extract
100g dark chocolate chips
50g desiccated coconut

These little balls of joy are incredibly tasty. With only a few ingredients, these are great to make in larger quantities as they freeze very well.

1 Blend the avocado in a food processor until it is very smooth. Add the protein powder, vanilla extract and almond extract and blend until mixed thoroughly.

2 Melt the chocolate chips in a heatproof bowl, either in short bursts in the microwave, stirring in between, or by suspending the bowl over a pan of simmering water.

3 Add the avocado mixture into the bowl of melted chocolate and stir until everything is well combined. Cover the bowl with cling film and chill for 2 hours.

4 Tip the desiccated coconut onto a small side plate. Scoop walnut-sized portions of the mixture and roll around in your hands to create even balls. You should be able to make 12. Roll each ball around in the coconut and place on some baking paper. Keep in the fridge for up to a week.

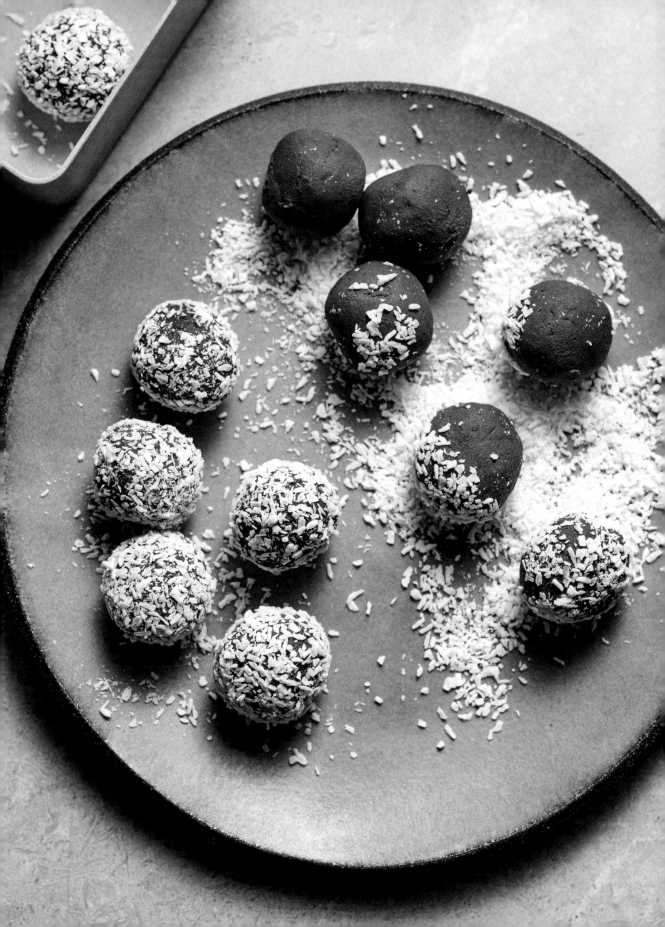

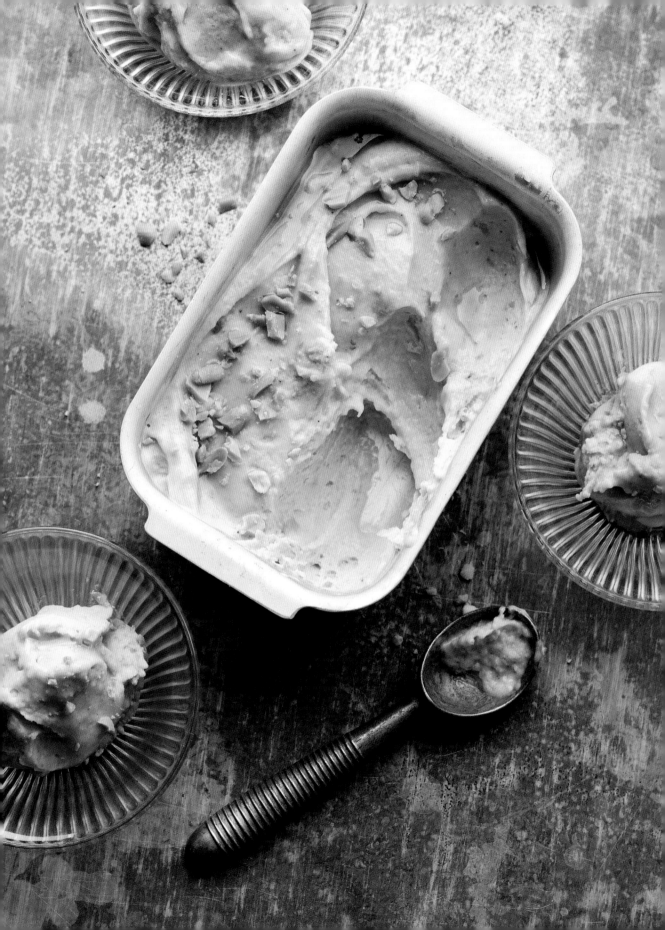

SOFT-SCOOP BANANA AND MAPLE ICE CREAM

PER SERVING | **225** CALS | **5G** PROTEIN | **7G** FAT | **35G** CARBS

prep
15 MINS +
FREEZING

FREEZE

SERVES 4

6 small or 5 medium
   bananas (you need about
   500g flesh once peeled)
50g roasted, salted
   peanuts
4 tbsp maple syrup

tip

*Make sure you get the ice
cream out of the freezer in
plenty of time before you
want to eat it, so it can
soften up again.*

*Everyone loves ice cream. I find this works best the riper
your bananas are. Don't throw those brown bananas away –
make ice cream instead.*

1 Peel the bananas and slice into rough chunks. Spread
them out on a tray and cover with cling film. Freeze at least
overnight until frozen solid. Roughly chop 10g of the peanuts
and set aside.

2 Tip the frozen banana into a food processor and blitz until
the banana is broken up into small pieces – it will look quite
crumbly at this point. Add 3 tbsp of the maple syrup to the
processor and keep blending until the mixture is smooth
and creamy.

3 Add 40g of the peanuts to the blender and pulse a few
times to incorporate them, but don't blend too much as
you want them in chunks.

4 You can spoon into bowls now and serve as a soft-set ice
cream. Top each bowl with a drizzle of the remaining maple
syrup and a quarter of the reserved chopped peanuts.
Alternatively, divide into small freezer-proof tubs and top
with the syrup and peanuts. Freeze until required, then
bring out of the freezer 10 minutes or so before eating
to soften a little.

204
CALS

SKINNY OREO SHAKE

PER SERVING | **204** CALS | **18G** PROTEIN | **6G** FAT | **21G** CARBS

prep
5 MINS   FREEZE

SERVES 2

250g fat-free cottage
   cheese
230ml skimmed milk,
   plus extra if needed
3 Oreo cookies, plus
   2 (optional) cookies,
   to serve
1 tsp powdered sweetener
1 tsp vanilla extract
low-fat squirty cream,
   to serve (optional)

tip

*I like this shake as it isn't
too sweet, but you can
add some no-calorie
sweetener to it, if you like.*

*I love milkshakes, however, they tend to be overly sweet and
sickly when bought from a shop. This is a great alternative
that isn't too sweet. Enjoy!*

1 In a blender or food processor, blitz the cottage cheese
until smooth – you may want to add a little of the milk to
assist the blending.

2 Add the remaining ingredients to the blender and blitz;
add a splash more milk if you like it a bit thinner, but remember
that it will thicken slightly when chilled.

3 Chill for around 1 hour before pouring into two glasses
and enjoying, or just keep in the fridge until ready to drink.

4 For an extra special treat, top each glass with a swirl
of low-fat squirty cream and an extra cookie.

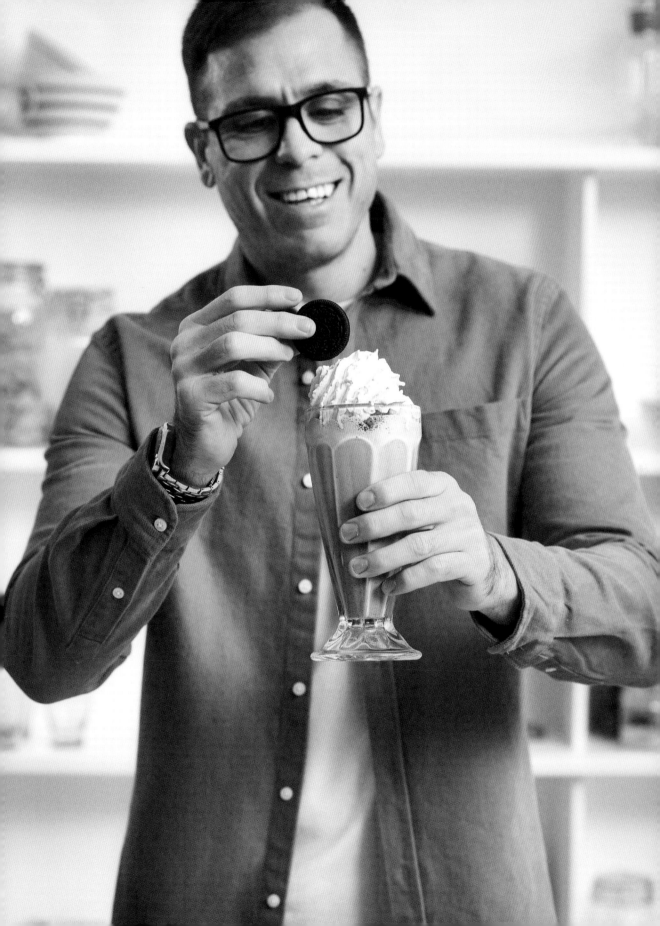

INDEX

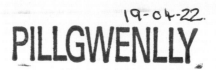

PILLGWENLLY

19-04-22.

Acknowledgements

I would like to thank all those closest to me who continue to support me, with a very special thank you to Charlotte and Frank in particular.

I'd like to thank my agent Charlie and all the crew who have worked on putting this book together – Emma & Alex, Jamie, Phil, Hannah, Becci, Ione, Paula and all at Michael Joseph.

I'd also like to give a shout to our fans and followers for trusting in us and helping us to make this possible. We owe a huge thank you to all those people.

And finally, I'd like to say a huge well done to all the people using our books to change their lifestyle and to those who have committed to change.

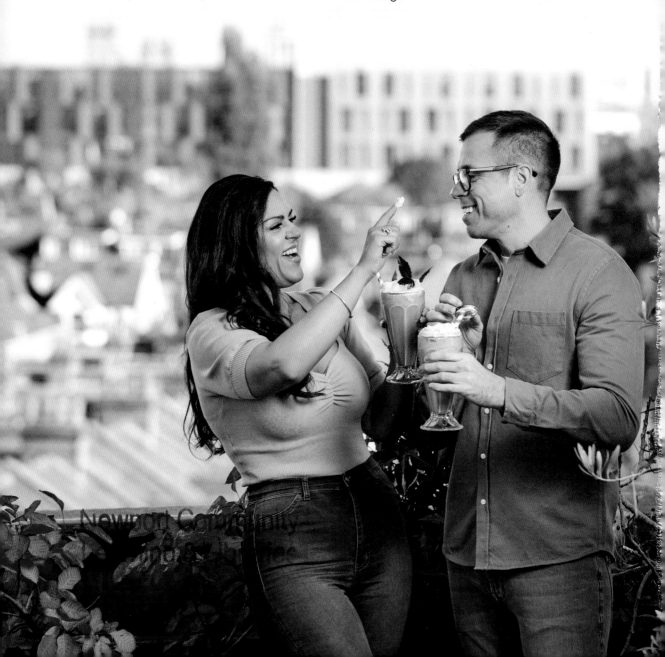